Mark R. Pitkin

Biomechanics for Life

Introduction to Sanomechanics

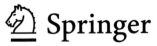 Springer

Author
Mark R. Pitkin, Ph.D., D.Sc.
Research Professor of Physical Medicine
and Rehabilitation
Tufts University School of Medicine
Boston, MA 02111
USA
and
Director of Center for Human Performance
New England Sinai Hospital
Stoughton, MA 02072
USA
mpitkin@tuftsmedicalcenter.org

ISBN 978-3-642-17176-5   e-ISBN 978-3-642-17177-2

DOI 10.1007/978-3-642-17177-2

Springer Heidelberg Dordrecht London New York

Library of Congress Control Number: 2011921939

© Springer-Verlag Berlin Heidelberg 2011

Cover design: eStudioCalamar, Figueres/Berlin

Printed on acid-free paper

Springer is part of Springer Science+Business Media (www.springer.com)

Biomechanics for Life

About the Author and the Book

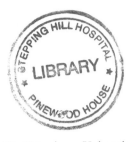

Dr. Pitkin graduated *Summa Cum Laude* from St. Petersburg University (Russia) in Mechanics. He received his Ph.D. from the Central Institute for Prosthetic Research, Moscow, and the Doctor of Technical Sciences (D.Sc.) degree from LETI University, St. Petersburg. Before joining the faculty of Tufts University, Dr. Pitkin headed the Foot Biomechanics Department at the St. Petersburg Institute of Prosthetics. He was a Visiting Scientist at the Human Performance Laboratory at The University of Calgary, and at the Newman Laboratory for Biomechanics and Human Rehabilitation at MIT. Dr. Pitkin's previous book, *Biomechanics of Lower Limb Prosthetics*, published by Springer in 2010, presents the results of his years of work in the field of mathematical and structural modeling. The book "serves as a foundation for designing and manufacturing contemporary lower limb prosthetics as an invaluable tool for prosthetic research" (*JAMA*, 2010; 304:21: http://jama.ama-assn.org/content/304/21/2418.extract).

In the current book, the reader will find a new approach to improving health. The author has called this approach "sanomechanics," from the Latin *sanus* (healthy) and *mechanicus* (science of the motion of bodies subjected to forces). The focus of sanomechanics is on exercising with an understanding of the biomechanical consequences of one's movements. This understanding is based on the author's theory of the floating skeleton, which postulates a hydraulic connection between synovial joints. The theory explains the greater or lesser success of any exercise, appealing to the ability of the human skeleton to absorb and transform forces and moments from the body segments and the environment. This ability vanishes with age and illness; and the deeper our understanding of the nature of how our skeleton functions, the better we will be able to improve, protect, and prolong our skeleton's health.

This book, with its multidisciplinary analysis of proven facts and new hypotheses, can be useful to researchers, practitioners, and students in the health professions, and to anyone who is interested in understanding the role of biomechanics in improving their well-being.

Preface

Physician, heal thyself
Luke 4:23

Until I was 47, I was generally healthy and considered myself to be quite athletic. I would jog two to three miles a couple of times a week; every other day I went to the gym, worked out with weights, and would finish with a swim and the sauna. I played tennis, skied, and hiked on vacations. My diet was what is considered healthy, I was not a smoker, and I didn't carry around any extra weight. This was the first period of my life.

At 47, I began experiencing an uncomfortable sensation in the balls of my feet whenever I walked. What was first a sensation grew more acute, and soon gradually transformed into pain at every step. A similarly painful sensation was developing in my wrists and fingers, which I couldn't flex without steadily increasing pain. I shared these new concerns with my doctor during my annual check-up, but on that day, like on a few lucky days, I had no pain in any of my joints, so I spoke in a lighthearted tone, smiling ashamedly, as if revealing guilt. Soon enough the pain returned, and after blood tests, X-rays, 2 weeks of Tylenol every 4 hours, and a list of medications of ascending strength and side effects, the first period of my life closed, and the second began.

Besides analgesics, the list of remedies considered and tried was long: physical therapy, acupuncture, massages, long swims, hypnosis, even mud therapy. Every 6 months, in the fall and in spring, I had to take several shots of Voltaren (diclofenac) to control the pain.

One day in yoga class, when all poses were painful as usual, I experienced a pleasant sensation while doing one of the exercises. It is the one where you lie on your back with both legs lifted at $90°$, and then slowly swing them to the floor, alternating on each side. The sensation, as I said, was pleasant, and I would have stayed in the pose longer, were it not for the instructor's command to move to the next pose. At the end of the session, I took account of my body's signals. My body had resisted all but one position by sending signals of discouragement in the form of pain. The only sensation of pleasure I received, then, must have been a signal of encouragement. And if encouragement, then the body wanted me to do something.

---

[1]Pitkin M (1993) Floating skeleton concept to explain causes of injuries in spine and success of any therapeutic procedure. In: Proceedings of the XIV International Conference on ISB, 1993, Paris, France, pp 1052–1053

But what? I think I've found it. I remembered a paper I had presented in 1993 at the Congress of the International Society of Biomechanics in Paris,[1] in which a possible answer lay hidden. In this book I've recorded my thoughts on why and how our bodies encourage and discourage us, and on how, by listening attentively to their signals, we can heal ourselves. Now, in the third period of my life, I am healing myself.

September 2010   Mark. R. Pitkin
Boston, MA, USA

Acknowledgments

I am grateful to my wife for her inspiration and to my son for critically reading the manuscript, and for consenting to demonstrate the sanomechanical exercises. I am pleased to acknowledge the New England Sinai Hospital in Stoughton, MA, and Tufts University School of Medicine in Boston, MA, for their longtime support of the Center for Human Performance where most of the biomechanical studies presented in the book were conducted. I am particularly grateful to my colleagues working at the Department of Orthopedics, Tufts University School of Medicine, for initiating the experimental verification of the floating skeleton concept.

Introduction

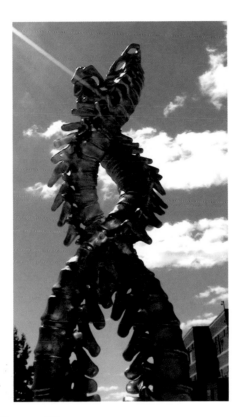

Double spine spiral (fragment).[2]

The *Double Spine Spiral* sculpture stands in front of New England Baptist Hospital in Brookline, MA, an institution renowned for orthopedic surgery. For me, it is a powerful reminder about the value of the long-lasting flexibility of the skeleton; the unfortunate alternative brings people to the Hospital.

---

[2]By Shelly Bradbury, New England Baptist Hospital, Brookline, MA.

People have always tried to prolong and enhance the skeleton's natural flexibility and health, and many training systems and philosophies have been developed to further that goal. Still, the number of patients at orthopedic hospitals is steadily increasing.

You will find in this book a new approach to improving your health through improving the well-being of your skeleton. I call this approach "sanomechanics™," from the Latin *sanus* (healthy) and *mechanicus* (science of motion of bodies subjected to forces). Sanomechanics can be thought of as mindful exercise, when you understand the mechanical origins and consequences of your actions. This understanding is based on my theory of the *floating skeleton* (Chap. 1) which explains the degree of success of any exercise you might have opted for in the past, or might now select. Though fitness and physical recovery systems are always introduced with a claim of novelty, their success – or lack of it – depends on whether or not they adhere to some common principles, mostly intuitive, which you will find in this book.

You will learn how to begin your day with several exercises, and will learn why these exercises are useful for maintaining good health, and how they help avoid unnecessary risks in everyday activities. Traditional biomechanics, after connecting to your active mind, will allow you to generate rational – and therefore powerful – autosuggestions for more positive results. You will adapt biomechanics, the respected academic discipline, to biomechanics for *your* life – *sanomechanics*.

In Chapter 1 the reader will become familiar with the *floating skeleton concept*, which was developed to better explain the biomechanics of the skeletal response to loads our bodies endure every day. The main scientific hypothesis is the existence of a hydraulic net component in the musculoskeletal system.

In Chapter 2 sanomechanics is defined as a discipline and as a new approach to exercising. It combines new techniques with autosuggestion and a specific "criterion of correctness."

Chapter 3, called "Biomechanics for Life" after the book's title, describes the biomechanical challenges with which our routine activities burden our skeleton. Ways to reduce these risks are discussed.

A detailed description of the sanomechanical series is presented in Chapter 4. Special attention is paid to the sanomechanical in-bed exercises, aimed at preparing the body for the dramatic changes in loads we experience when transitioning from the horizontal to the vertical position every morning.

Chapter 5 is devoted to the theoretical and practical aspects of obtaining and analyzing data on kinematics and dynamics of locomotion. Basic principles of modeling the human body for motion analysis and related equipment are considered. The phenomenon of ballistic synergy in gait is examined along with the phenomena of resonance and anti-resonance. These help us appreciate the involvement of the musculoskeletal system not only in load bearing, but also in the sophisticated and still not well understood hierarchy of motor control. If you find the material of this chapter too technical, it can be skipped without compromising the understanding of other material in the book.

Some elements of biomechanics of respiration with a focus on exercises for clearing the airways can be found in Chapter 6. The reader will see that although the material is only remotely related to the skeleton, the approach to the exercises is still sanomechanical. This is the practicality of the methodology of sanomechanics. Hopefully, the reader will be able to develop a new series of exercises to meet his particular needs. If this happens, the author will consider his mission accomplished.

Contents

Floating Skeleton Concept

1

The fetal skeleton floats, entirely immersed in fluid contained inside of a flexible shell. As the fetus develops, the periosteum tightens around the bones, and the joints are covered by capsules filled with synovial fluid. We believe that even in adolescents and adults, all synovial joints are hydraulically connected with each other, forming a distinctive morphological and physiological system. We will present the arguments and the facts supporting the *floating skeleton* concept, and will show the biomechanical advantages of the newly postulated anatomical system.

1.1
Borelli's Biomechanics and Its Limitations

Since rotation is a major type of motion in the human muscular-skeletal system, it is no surprise that the beginning of contemporary biomechanics as a science was associated with a detailed application of the concept of *moments*. The *moment* of a force is a measure of its tendency to rotate an object about a given point or axis. The moment is defined as the rotational potential of the forces acting on a joint. During balance or rotation with constant angular velocity, the resultant moment M_r of forces causing rotation at angle φ equals the resultant moment M_a of forces providing resistance to that rotation (Fig. 1.1). In accelerated angular motion, M_r is greater than M_a, and their exact difference is given by Newton's second law for rotation:

$$M_r - M_a = I\ddot{\varphi} \tag{1.1}$$

where I is the moment of inertia of the rotating link, and $\ddot{\varphi}$ is its angular acceleration.

Muscles affecting a joint's articulation, the force of gravity, and ground reactions may contribute either to M_a or to M_r, depending on the body's configuration during different phases of locomotion. In gait, for example, during most of the stance phase, foot plantarflexors provide resistance (M_a) to dorsiflexion rotation in the ankle, and after heel rise, they cause active plantarflexion (M_r). The same is true for the body weight mg and ground reaction vector R, since these forces change orientation relative to the joint's center from anterior to posterior several times during a stride (Winter 1979; Perry 1992).

M.R. Pitkin, *Biomechanics for Life*,
DOI: 10.1007/978-3-642-17177-2_1, © Springer-Verlag Berlin Heidelberg 2011

Fig. 1.1 Resultant moment M_r of forces causing rotation at the angle φ and resultant moment M_a of forces providing resistance to that rotation. Reactions in the joint are not counted since their lever arms relative to the joint equal zero

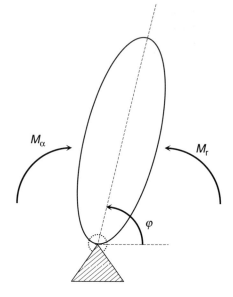

In biomechanics, the concept of the moment is used to describe the relationship between forces generated by muscles and the resultant motions. It was first described by the Italian scientist Giovanni Alfonso Borelli, in the manuscript *De Motu Animalium* (Borelli 1680) published in Rome after his death. Borelli showed that the levers of the musculoskeletal system - not force - magnify motion (Fig. 1.2), and determine the position of the body's center of gravity. Borelli made a significant step toward applying mechanics to understanding human motion. Contemporary Borelli-like models of the musculoskeletal system represent the skeleton as a poly-linker with pin joints between solid links (Nordin et al. 1987). Such poly-linker models are behind the Lagrange equations used today for computerized motion analysis systems. One can calculate tension in muscles, ligaments, and bones, assuming the constraints of solid mechanics.

However, when calculating forces and moments with these systems, a simple poly-linker model does not adequately model reality (Simon 2004). For example, the Borelli-like models cannot explain sudden injury caused by routine loads, when similar or smaller loads had been previously accepted by the body for thousands of cycles.

1.2
Loads and Pressures Applied to Joint Heads

Calculations of forces in joints in vivo can be evaluated indirectly or directly. For indirect measurements, computerized *motion analysis systems* are used (Chap. 5). The systems, such as the *Vicon Motion Analysis System*,[1] collect optical data and ground reactions during locomotion, and then process them with the Newton/Lagrange equations. The equations

---

[1]Vicon Motion Systems, Inc., Centennial, CO

Fig. 1.2 Borelli's diagram of forces and moments generated by muscles and gravity (Borelli 1680). With permission from Museo Galileo - Institute and Museum of the History of Science, Florence. Photo by Eurofoto

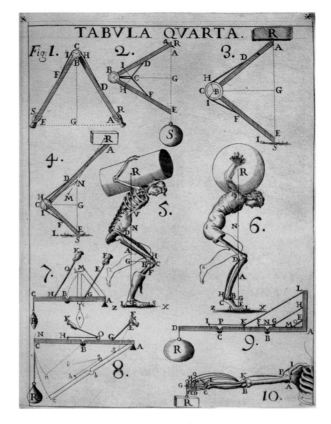

are developed using the representation of the body as system of solids connected with 2D or 3D pivotal joints, as suggested by Borelli (1680).

To estimate the pressures on the joint heads, one needs to divide the applied force by the area of contact between the two joint heads. Pressure p is a measure of contact of two bodies and is defined as

$$p = \frac{F}{S} \tag{1.2}$$

where F is the contact force and S is the contact area.

In biomechanics, pressure is investigated in two realms. First, it is the analysis of how the human body interacts with the environment, such as the ground, sports equipment, shoes, furniture and tools. Pressure is also analyzed in the biomechanics of limb prosthetics. The second area is the analysis of pressure inside the body: in liquids, organs, vessels, and joints. It is pressure and its distribution, not the generating force itself, which causes pain and leads to injuries, which is why interest in its study arose.

When presented with a calculated value of pressure, it is good to know how F and S were measured, and whether under dynamic or static conditions. Since we are looking for the cause of pain in joints, we need to discuss here what is known about joint forces and joint contact areas.

1.2.1
Pressure in Statics

During one-legged standing, the talar surface of the ankle joint is loaded with the weight of the part of the body positioned above it. The weight acting on the ankle joint is equal to the body weight minus the weight of the foot.

On average, the weight of a foot is 1.5% of the body weight (Winter 1991). Therefore, while standing on one leg, the talar surface of the ankle joint must withstand 98.5% of the body weight. With the gravitational constant $g = 9.81 \, \text{m} / \text{s}^2$ and a man's mass taken to be $m = 75 \, \text{kg}$, he will weigh $P = mg = 75 \cdot 9.81 = 736 \, \text{N}$. Consequently, the head of the talar head will be loaded with $P_1 = 736 \cdot 0.985 = 725 \, \text{N}$.

Thus, in calculating the pressure in the ankle joint using Eq. 1.2, we already know the expression's numerator F, which will be P_1. The methodology for obtaining the value of P_1 requires only a skillful dissection of cadavers, and a set of scales for measuring the weights of the cadavers' parts. The estimate we just made for P_1 could have been made hundreds of years ago, even before Newton's Laws. Not so for the expression's denominator S. The in vivo estimates of contact areas in the joints have become available only recently, thanks to the development of computerized imaging technologies. In a study of real-time in vivo cartilage contact deformation in the ankle joint (Li et al. 2008), the contact area was estimated as a function of time along the loading history, using a combined magnetic resonance imaging (MRI) and dual-orthogonal fluoroscopic imaging technique. Ankle images shown in Fig. 1.3a were digitized to reproduce the contours of the tibia, the talus, and their cartilage surfaces, as shown in Fig. 1.3b. The subject lifted his right foot and loaded his left ankle. The contact area increased from $150.2 \pm 122.1 \, \text{mm}^2$ in the first second, to $377.2 \pm 84.0 \, \text{mm}^2$ after 300 s of loading. Location of the contact area did not change, as shown in Fig. 1.4.

If we take the results of this study as an estimate of the area S in Eq. 1.2 and combine it with our estimate for P_1, then we will get an interval of pressure P_t on the talar cartilage of 1.9 to 4.8 MPa. With what known interfaces can that interval of pressure be compared? According to

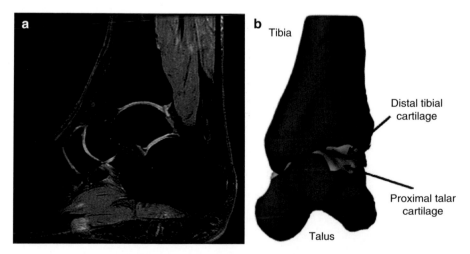

Fig. 1.3 (**a**) A typical sagittal plane MRI of the ankle joint; (**b**) the 3D ankle joint model constructed using the 3D MRIs of the ankle joint (From Li et al. (2008). With permission from Elsevier)

Fig. 1.4 Compressive cartilage contact deformation distributions on the tibial cartilage surface at different time intervals after loading (From Li et al. (2008). With permission from Elsevier)

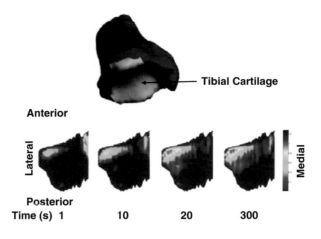

Thompson and Sorvig (Thompson and Sorvig 2008), the pressure exerted by a bulldozer or military tank on the ground is about 0.55 MPa, while the pressure under a woman's stiletto heel can be over 13 MPa. The estimate for p_t was obtained for standing subjects; in gait or running the pressure would be up to three times greater, because of the corresponding rise in the vertical component of the ground reaction, which is represented by P_i in Eq. 1.2. We can conclude that the pressure on the talar and tibial cartilages is close to that under women's spiked heels. Is this big or small? The answer is quite obvious to those unfortunate men whose feet have experienced a terrible hit from a stiletto heel. For others, it will be sufficient to notice the deep pockmarks in parquet.

1.2.2
Pressures in Dynamics

A sound person does not "feel" loads on the feet or the skeletal joints during routine activities. All this changes when we are injured. Any muscle or ligament strain or joint injury immediately "informs" about the timing and magnitude of the muscle or ligament's contribution to the activity. The information is conveyed through pain, the body's signal to discourage its master from performing or continuing the movement, and "advice" to search for compensatory movements, which may be less painful.

We should conclude that sensory information, for example about gait, is misleading. A sound leg does not feel body weight, even though the sensitivity of the plantar surface of the foot is similar to the sensitivity of the palm of the hand. To demonstrate this phenomenon, one may ask a subject in a standing position to alternate between standing on one foot and two feet. Then ask if he/she feels a significant difference in the load applied to the leg, and specifically to the supporting foot. More likely, the answer will be "no big difference if any in the feeling of the load applied to the foot." While the answer is quite typical, it should surprise and warn us, since the actual difference in the load is as big as one half of the body weight. We see from this experiment how signals that fall within the boundaries of a safe zone of loading are filtered.

The boundaries themselves are task dependent. Ask your subject, while he stands on one foot, to bend his leg and hold his ankle with his hand, so that the foot's plantar surface faces up. Now, apply a small weight (a book, for example) to the plantar surface of the lifted foot. Now put another book on top of the first. The subject will easily distinguish the weight of one book from the weight of two books. This is the same foot of the same subject who did not "feel" the difference between one half of his body weight and his full body weight.

Physiology refers to this phenomenon of selective feedback as the principle of minimum of afferent information (van Dijk 1979; Schneidman et al. 2003). The principle states that for repetitive, routine, and automotive or well-known movements, the body tries to minimize the flow of nerve signals from the periphery to the center (afferent information). The rationale is to relieve the brain from routine signal processing, to allow it to more effectively process an abruptly large quantity of afferent information in case of emergency. An example of such an emergency is when a walker realizes just before his swinging leg is ready to touch the ground ("heel-on" event of the gait cycle), that the ground is slippery and landing at the predetermined spot is dangerous and must be avoided. The motor control system rapidly switches from automotive to custom mode and develops a program for either a larger step or for a jump over the dangerous area.

Loads during locomotion play a dual role for the joints. They may cause wear of the contacting surfaces, but they may also stimulate their recovery and development. If the recovery process is at least in balance with the process of wear and tear of the cartilages in the joints, we do not need to feel our weight during locomotion, and we do not. If the balance shifts in the direction of deterioration, pain comes as a request to lower the loads. We see this in the elderly, as their cartilages are damaged faster than they can recover.

While the principle of minimum of afferent information offers an explanation for why self-analysis of sound gait is not an easy and straightforward task, it does not bring us any closer to an effective self-evaluation of the loads applied to specific joints. We need to look for objective methods, including the Borelli biomechanics, even with their known limitations.

If we want to estimate the loads applied to joints when walking, the simple calculation made above under static conditions does not suffice. Calculating the loads in dynamics of locomotion requires a combination of a mathematical model of the body in motion, hardware for collecting the input data, and software to make calculations according to the mathematical model within a reasonable timeframe. Though the mathematical modeling was developed about 100 years ago, effective hardware and computer software for data acquisition and *real-time* analysis became available only around the 1980s. This concept is discussed in greater details in Chap. 5, where the typical structure of computerized motion analysis systems is presented.

Here, I am showing a portion of a computer-generated report of a normal gait trial that pertains to loads in the ankle, knee and hip joints of the right leg during stance phase (from heel-on until toe-off). The chart on the left side of Fig. 1.5 contains a graph of the vertical Ground Reaction Force (GRF) plotted with a dotted line and the vertical components of the forces acting on the ankle (red line), knee (blue line), and hip (dashed line). The horizontal axis shows time normalized by duration of the stride period (from heel-on until heel-on of the same leg). The normalized time is expressed in percentages.

In the picture on the right side of Fig. 1.5, there is a skeletal lower body model, created with Vicon Motion Analysis System software. Depicted is the moment when the subject lands on the front force plate with his right foot (red), and his left foot (yellow) has almost broken contact with the back force plate. The blue arrow is a 3D visualization of the GRF vector, with its positioning corresponding to the so-called "load acceptance event" (Perry 1992) and marked with the vertical green line in the chart.

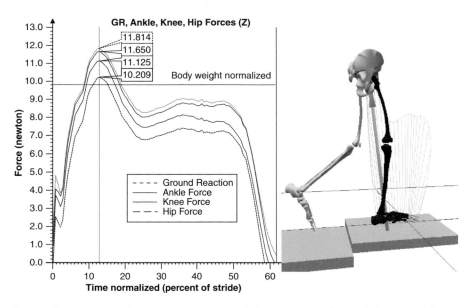

Fig. 1.5 Comparison of the vertical component of the ground reaction and the vertical forces applied to the ankle, knee and hip joints. Normalized body weight is indicated by the horizontal line. Data obtained during contact of the right leg (in *red*) with Kistler force plate shown in the Vicon movie window on the right (New England Sinai Hospital Center for Human Performance, Stoughton, MA)

The relationship between the weight P of a subject measured in Newtons, and mass m measured in kilograms is determined by Newton's second law as

$$P = mg \tag{1.3}$$

where $g = 9.81 \, \text{m} / \text{s}^2$ is the gravitational constant.

For ease of interpretation, the subject's weight P (1.3) was normalized by dividing it by the subject's mass m. A normalized force with a numerical value of g corresponds to the subject's full body weight. Values on the vertical axis are forces in Newtons, normalized by m. The body weight is marked on the chart by a horizontal line labeled as "Body weight normalized."

We can see from the numerical labels on the chart that 0.125 sec after heel-on (12.7% of stride period), the vertical component of the GRF reached 11.814N or 120.4% of the subject's weight. For the absolute value of the force applied to the talus head in the ankle joint we have 11.650N or 118.5% of the subject's weight. In the knee joint the force is 11.125N or 113.40%, and in the hip joint the force is 10.209N or 104.1%.

The graphs show that all the forces exceed the subject's body weight at the load acceptance event of the stance period while the second maxima are slightly smaller than the weight. This is the typical double-peak pattern first recorded by Elftman with a dynamographic platform (Elftman 1938), which is the prototype for the force plates in contemporary gait laboratories.

If we assume that the contact area in the knee joint is within the range estimated for the ankle joint (Li et al. 2008), then for the subjects with weight $P = 736$ N the peak pressures on the tibia head will range from 3.7 to 5.3 MPa. This estimate is in agreement with the direct *in vivo* measurements of pressures on normal human acetabular cartilage that were collected from implanted instrumented femoral head hemiprostheses (Morrell et al. 2005). Even with such high pressures, the loading of the joint in dynamics may be less damaging than in statics for two related reasons. First, there is no continuous loading on the same area as in statics. Second, the high loading lasts for a short time (about 0.1 s), with 0.9 s used for recuperation of the cartilages before loading at the next step.

Another source of knowledge about actual loads on the joint-contacting surfaces is the direct measurement of pressures in implanted artificial joints. In the first such study, contact pressure within the implanted hip joint was investigated (Hodge et al. 1986). The pressures were measured in vivo by a telemetric system embedded in the metal sphere of the artificial femoral head. The pressure was recorded at ten discrete locations. Data were acquired during surgery, recovery, rehabilitation, and normal activity, for more than 1 year after surgery. During level gait, the peak local pressure at one of the locations reached 6.78 MPa, and was almost twice as large during transition from sitting to standing. This range was consistent with the cadaver studies designed for deferent simulated phases of gait cycles and verified with a finite element model (Anderson et al. 2008).

Studies of the porous structure of cartilage suggest that such high pressures are withstood in anatomical joints hydraulically by the fluid film in the cartilage, which distributes pressure. The cartilage becomes compressed under the load, and fluid is exuded from the saturated cartilage layer. This fluid film takes some of the load from the cartilage tissues, thus preserving the cartilage's integrity (Fick et al. 2010). The directional dependence of the pore structure, also known as anisotropy, allows cartilage to deform without significantly altering the axial porosity of the matrix even at very large strains (Greene et al. 2008).

While a consensus exists on the hydraulic protection of the joint's contacting surfaces, an important question has to be raised: can the small volume of synovial liquid in a single joint be sufficient to mitigate the high pressure exerted on the joint?

1.3
New Hypothetical Protective Structure

When I first made this estimate for pressures in statics and dynamics it was hard for me to believe that human cartilage can sustain such enormous pressures, considering that when we walk or run, the loads are cyclic and occur thousands of times. With all due respect and admiration to our body for its ability to recover, regenerate, and repair small damages in tissues, the pressures of 4–8 MPa magnitude seemed to be too massive for biological objects like human cartilages. I began thinking about the existence of an unknown structure in the musculoskeletal system that, in addition to the small amounts of synovial liquid in the joint capsules, protects the joints' heads from destructive pressures. When working efficiently, that structure would have to decrease the peak pressures to a safer level. When that hypothetical structure goes out of order, the pressures would be as high as we just calculated above, and a series of well-known pathological events could occur.

However, as far as I know, there are no additional elements within the musculoskeletal system to which such a powerful structure can be attributed. Therefore, a reasonable possibility would be a new combination of already known elements producing the effect of interest. That combination, as I will discuss below, could be fluid + periosteum, which forms a hydraulic net of the synovial joints.

1.4
Floating Skeleton Concept

Most of the body's joints are diarthrodial, which means their articulation is freely movable. In a diarthrodial joint, the contiguous bony surfaces are covered with articular cartilage, and connected by ligaments lined by a synovial membrane (Gray and Lewis, 1918). It has been a general convention that the synovial liquid is contained inside the synovial membrane, as illustrated in Fig. 1.6.

Before presenting the *floating skeleton concept*, we will need to talk about one more component of the musculoskeletal system, namely the *periosteum*. The periosteum is a membrane that covers the outer surface of all bones. The inner layer of the periosteum (cambium layer) contains progenitor cells that develop into osteoblasts, and which are responsible for increasing the width and the overall size of the bone. The periosteum is attached to the bone by strong collagenous fibers, and is also attached to muscles and tendons.

The *floating skeleton concept* proposed by the author (Pitkin 1993) stipulates that the joint capsules form a net of hydraulically connected containers. Due to the hydraulic connectivity of the capsules, the synovial fluid transmits extra pressure equally to each of them. The hydraulic connection between the capsules is made possible by a layer of fluid between the periosteum and bone surface. In light of the importance of the intimate connection between the cambium layer of the periosteum and the bone, the liquid layer might not cover the entire outer surface of the bone. Certain canals might be connecting the synovial containers. Even a thin film or canal would be sufficient to connect joints hydraulically.

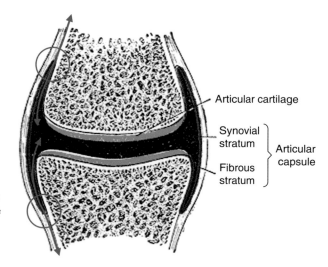

Fig. 1.6 Typical diarthroidal joint (Modified from Gray and Lewis. (1918) with permission from Bartleby. com, Inc.). *Orange arrows* over circled zones indicate the hypothesized permeation of synovial fluid from the capsule through the fibrous stratum, filling the space between the bone and periosteum

Articular cartilage

Synovial stratum }
Fibrous stratum } Articular capsule

Because some muscle fibers are attached to the periosteum, they pull the periosteum away from the bone's surface when they are activated. If the attachment zone is located around the network canal postulated above, the pulling away of the periosteum will pump and spread the fluid from the surrounding synovial capsules.

The dispersion of the fluid between the periosteum and the bone's outer surface can also be explained via capillarity, osmosis, or both mechanisms. Capillary action, which is essential for transmission of blood, lymph, saliva, nasal mucus, and tears, is not dependent on excesses of pressure, and is capable of anti-gravitational fluid delivery (Batchelor 1967).

1.4.1
Arguments Supporting the Floating Skeleton Concept

Before we discuss the direct evidence of the floating skeleton, let us consider some indirect supporting data from studies focused on other topics. The sub-periosteum fluid can be found in the cambial layer of the periosteum (Squier et al. 1990). Fluid under the periosteum shell along the tubular bones can be seen in an X-ray from a study (Leroy et al. 2009) of an 8-month-old girl with Mucolipidosis II (ML II) (Fig. 1.7). Hers is a case of I-cell disease, which is a slowly progressive inborn error of metabolism. An outline of periosteal margins called "periosteal cloaking" is seen here in the humerus and forearm bones. This unique phenomenon is transient, disappearing by age 18 months, and cannot be easily observed in normal children and adults. Thus, it would be a challenge to demonstrate visually the hydraulic connectivity of the joints *in vivo*.

An increase in the amount of liquid in a joint due to injury or infection or other type of joint structure is called joint *effusion*. It is usually associated with an increase in the volume of the joint capsule called distention, and inhibition of the musculature surrounding the joint. This is thought to be a reflectory mechanism that constrains the joint's

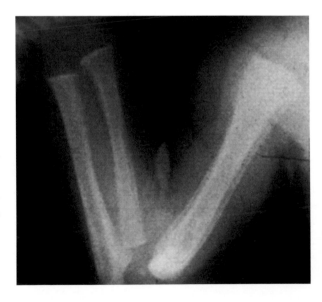

Fig. 1.7 "Periosteal cloaking," seen here in the humerus and forearm bones of an 8-month-old girl and often observed in infants with Mucolipidosis II (ML II) (Adapted from Leroy et al. (2009). With permission from GeneReviews, http://www.genetests.org; Copyright, University of Washington, Seattle 1997–2010)

participation in locomotion during its healing, and protects the joint from further damage if the level of its activity remains as before the injury (Hopkins, Ingersoll et al. 2001; Palmieri-Smith, Kreinbrink et al. 2007). Simultaneously, pain emerges as a notification about need to limit the joint's activity.

Let us assume that before the injury, the joint was hydraulically connected with the entire skeletal net. Then how should the body begin the healing process after the injury? Just as patients are quarantined during an outbreak to protect the uninfected, the first step prior to effusion and distention should be to seal off the involved capsule, isolating it from the net. Once hydraulically isolated, the joint's heads no longer share their pressure with the net, and become subjected to the stiletto-like forces calculated before. If we load these joints during the period of isolation, we risk compromising recovery after injury. Therefore, the occurrence of pain is biomechanically justified as a means of discouraging those movements that exert excessive pressures on the joint's heads.

1.4.2
Floating Versus Hydraulic

Here we want to make a distinction between the terms *hydraulic* and *floating* with respect to the skeleton. The first is applied to the concept of soft tissues and organs containing fluids and forming specific containers supporting the trunk angulations. An example is given in Fig. 1.8 showing an abdominal fluid ball comprised of internal organs (Bartelink 1957). When compressed by the spine, ribs, and abdominal muscles while the trunk is bent, it generates the counter forces that help stabilize the trunk and extend it further. Thus, the hydraulics of body cavities in mammals serve a supporting function to the bony skeleton, and this contribution is associated in the literature with the term *hydraulic skeleton* (Lunkenheimer and Ising 1974; Barra et al. 2004). The practicality of the hydraulic skeleton concept has been confirmed in rehabilitation and prevention of trauma. Athletes are recommended to wear wide belts and tighten them before lifting heavy weights (Granata et al. 1997). The biomechanics of the supportive ball is based on an application of Laplace's law, which considers tension in the wall of the ball, its curvature, and pressure inside the ball (Michael and Sircar 2010). Most other applications of fluid mechanics in relation to understanding how the human body functions have focused on the analysis of biofluid flow (Grotberg and Jensen 2004).

The term *hydraulic skeleton* is also used in the analysis of the locomotion of insects (Casey 1991) or architecture of trees and other plants (Tyree and Frank 1992; Sack et al. 2003). A hydraulic skeleton functions by the inflation of compression-resisting fluid under pressure. Some of these hydraulic structures, like mammalian penises, are inflated by muscle contractions that force fluid into the container. Other hydraulic skeletons, such as embryonic notochords,[2] are inflated osmotically (Koehl et al. 2000). Delivery of fluid to the flexible containers is a mechanism of force-generation. It controls their shape, and permits them to stiffen and straighten to resist the compressing and bending external loads.

---

[2]Notochord: Greek *noton* back + *chorde* cord: a longitudinal flexible rod of cells that in embryos of the higher vertebrates forms the supporting axis of the body

Fig. 1.8 Diagram to suggest how the abdominal fluid ball, attached to the costal margin, would provide some support for the upper trunk, in case of lifting with the trunk flexed forward (Adapted from Bartelink (1957). With permission and copyright © of the British Editorial Society of Bone and Joint Surgery)

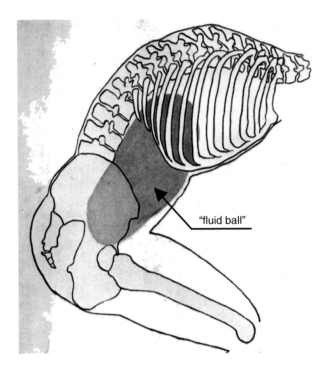

"fluid ball"

Therefore, when talking about the bony skeleton immersed in the fluid between the bones' outer surfaces and the periosteum sheath (shell), we prefer using the term *floating* introduced elsewhere (Pitkin 1993).

1.4.3
Archimedes Force Decreases Pressure on Joint Cartilages

All body segments and organs operate in the gravitational field. When an object is submerged in liquid, its interaction with its environment is determined by the fact that both the object and the liquid are under the effect of gravity. As a result, when an object is submerged in liquid, the buoyant force is applied to it. The force acts against the gravitational force, and is equal to the weight of the liquid displaced by the object (Archimedes' Law). There are two reasons for the phenomenon of buoyancy: fluid pressure increases with depth, and is exerted in all directions (Pascal principle). When an object is positioned in a container filled with liquid, the upward force that is applied to the submerged object affects the interface between the object and the bottom of the container.

Imagine a container A with object B, which presses on resilient ball C, as shown in panel 1 of Fig. 1.9. The diagram depicts the deformed shape of the ball under the weight of object B. Now let liquid be poured into container A (panel 2 of Fig. 1.9). The resilient ball C will now experience a smaller compression. The portion of the object B that remains submerged in the liquid will be determined by the buoyant force. The amount of this force will be equal to the weight of the liquid displaced by the portion of the object B that is submerged in the liquid. Since the buoyant force acts in the direction opposite to the gravitational force, its value will be subtracted from the weight of the object B when calculating the force B exerts on C. Consequently, a smaller force will compress ball C, and the deformation of the ball will be smaller than in a container without liquid.

Now we illustrate the difference between the traditional understanding of separate joint capsules and the floating skeleton concept. Figure 1.10 schematically depicts a portion of the leg skeleton along with the knee and ankle joints, whose synovial capsules are hydraulically disconnected. In Fig. 1.10, the layer of liquid between the bones and the periosteum connects both capsules.

If object B in Fig. 1.9 simulates skeletal bones in Fig. 1.10, container A simulates the periosteum, and ball C simulates joint cartilages, we will have an idea about the different

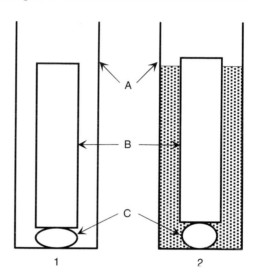

Fig. 1.9 Effect of buoyancy on compression in the container: 1 - object B in container A compresses resilient ball C; 2 - water is poured into the container, and the buoyant force acting on the object B decreases compression of the ball C

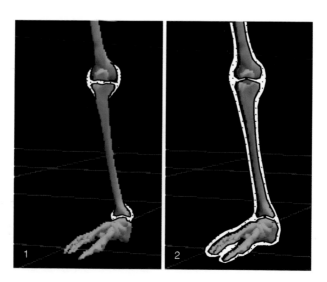

Fig. 1.10 Hydraulically isolated (1) and connected joints (2)

compressive loads acting on the cartilages in these two joints. Indeed, if the buoyant force is applied to the bones above a joint, the compressive load to the joint cartilage will be decreased by the weight of the synovial liquid in the volume of these bones.

1.4.4
Effect of Surface Tension and Capillarity

Capillarity is a phenomenon based on the surface-tension effect. The phenomenon is illustrated by putting a partially submerging thin tube (capillary) in water, perpendicularly to the surface. If the capillary is made out of a hydrophilic material like glass, the level of water in the capillary will be higher than the water level in the surrounding container.

The model we considered in Fig. 1.9 did not take into account the surface-tension effect that to some extent violates Archimedes' law of buoyancy (Falkovich et al. 2005). "Violation" means that the buoyant force will be smaller or greater, depending on whether the material of object B is hydrophilic or hydrophobic. Since cortical bone is hydrophilic, the buoyant force in the skeleton model in Fig. 1.10b, will be slightly decreased. Nevertheless, an adjustment to the value of Archimedes' buoyant force due to capillarity effect does not nullify Archimedes' law itself. In the field of gravity, even in a very thin column of liquid, pressure at its bottom will still be higher than at its top, which is the cause for the buoyant force's existence.

Therefore, the contribution of Archimedes' buoyant force to the reduction of the loads to joint cartilages has to be viewed as an additional mechanism in their lifelong protection.

1.4.5
Tension in the Walls of a Flexible Tube Filled with Water

Osmosis causes the vacuoles in a notochord to swell. This process is resisted by the sheath, and the internal pressure of the notochord consequently rises. As a result, the notochord elongates and straightens. The high density of the sheath plays a critical role in the notochord's elongation by providing counterpressure to the rising pressure inside. This becomes evident in the later stages of embryonic development, when collagenase digestion removes the sheath, and the flexural stiffness of the notochord is notably reduced. The sheathless notochord cannot push effectively on the surrounding embryonic tissues and folds up like a wet noodle (Koehl et al. 2000).

Substantial attention has been paid to investigating the deformation of flexible tubes filled with biofluids, like blood vessels (Grotberg and Jensen 2004), but it was Alexander who examined the deformation of such tubes that have skeletal structures inside (Alexander 1968). In particular, it was demonstrated that longer tubes filled with water are more flexible compared to shorter tubes.

A morphometric study of collagen orientations in the periosteum (Foolen et al. 2008) demonstrated that collagen fibers align with the preferential directions of long bone growth. The diaphyseal (middle part of the long bone) periosteum contained longitudinally oriented collagen fibers, while the collagen network of the epiphyseal part (bone heads) was randomly oriented. The authors explain that anisotropy by the particularities of bone growth. These data, when coupled with data about the orientation of the fibers in notochords (Koehl et al. 2000), and with greater flexibility of longer tubes (Alexander 1987; Koehl et al. 2000) may explain why the hydraulic component of the skeleton becomes activated only after a certain amount of bending in the joint. That is important for motion of the body segments when articulation in joints has to be either free or restricted. In gait, for example, a certain sequence of free and limited mobility in the ankle, knee, and hip joints forms a ballistic synergy, which is an attribute of normality in locomotion (Pitkin 2009).

According to our hypothesis, a hydraulically connected net of joint capsules constitutes an elastic shell that absorbs and distributes the extra pressure caused by the changing configuration of solid elements placed inside the shell. The simplest model of the floating skeleton consists of two rods elastically connected by an extension spring (Fig. 1.11a). The type of relative motion of the rod-contacting surfaces is cycloidal rolling without slipping (Fig. 1.11b). The rods are totally covered by an elastic shell with fluid in the space between the shell and the rods. The middle part of the shell represents a typical joint capsule.

Consider the articulation zones of the model (Fig. 1.12). In Zone A the modulus of the articulation angle corresponds to the joint's free movement or joint articulation without significant muscle control. Inside of that zone the major types of locomotional performances take place. Zones B+ and B− correspond to the range of motion during which there is possible braking with both active muscles and passive ligaments involved. Curvature change of the capsule due to joint articulation (Fig. 1.11) creates the extra inner pressure p_i of the fluid, as determined by Laplace's Law.

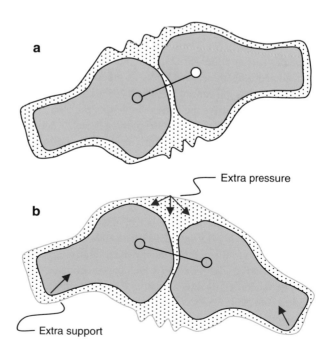

Extra pressure

Extra support

Fig. 1.11 Model of bending in the floating skeleton: (**a**) neutral position; (**b**) deformed position

Fig. 1.12 Zones of articulation in a typical joint. A, unrestricted mobility with neutral sensation; B− and B+, zones of restricted mobility with sensation of pleasure; C− and C+, zones of restricted mobility with sensation of pain

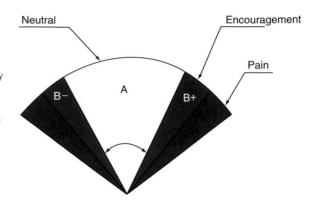

The pressure is transmitted (Pascal's Law), and creates additional force F_r of resistance to bending:

$$F_r = \left(p_e - p_i \right) \cdot S \tag{1.4}$$

where p_e is external pressure, and S is the area of the entire periosteum shell (Pitkin 1993). Resistance to bending rises in zones C+ and C−, where the continuation of bending generates pain, which signals the limit of articulation that is dangerous for the joint's integrity.

1.4.6
Tendon–Bone Connection

Muscles act on bones through tendons. The attachment of a tendon to the bone can be considered with increasing levels of precision. The simplest model of the tendon–bone connection was introduced by Borelli (1680). In that model, the tension of a rope generates a moment that rotates the bone relative to a pin joint. The model allowed Borelli to demonstrate that the mechanical outcome of a muscle's action depends not only on the tension generated, but also on a lever arm (a perpendicular from the point of rotation to the muscle's line of action).

Recent morphological studies show a very complex combination of tissues and anatomical formations in the zone where the tendon is attached to the bone. That zone is called the *enthesis*, and its investigation is so important for understanding the development of arthritis and trauma prevention that the concept of an *enthesis organ* was suggested (Benjamin and McGonagle 2001). The authors of the concept consider a collection of tissues adjacent to the enthesis itself, which jointly serve the common function of stress dissipation, and conditions under which that function can be compromised with extra loads.

The tendon or ligament attaches either directly to the bone or indirectly to it via the periosteum (Milz et al. 2005; Benjamin and McGonagle 2009). In both cases, dense fibrous connective tissue connects the tendon/ligament to the periosteum and provides the pull-away effect when the muscles are activated. Assuming that the floating skeleton concept is valid, we can attribute to the pull-away action of the tendons towards the periosteum not only the means for stress dissipation at the enthesis, but also the mechanism for pumping liquid through the space between the periosteum and the bone.

In ultrastructural studies on the enthesis of a rat's Achilles tendon (Rufai et al. 1996), it was found that certain cartilage (sesamoid and periosteal fibrocartilage) was covered with a layer of acellular, electron-dense material. This covering formed an articular surface layer, preventing direct contact between the cartilage and the surrounding cavity. The study offers possible evidence in favor of the hydraulic connection between synovial capsules through canals under the periosterum.

1.4.7
What If the Hydraulic Connection Is Broken?

Now we can discuss a pathological situation. When the hydraulic connection is broken and a joint is separated from the net, the joint's shock absorption capacity decreases in proportion to the area of the separated part of the net. After passing the safety threshold, the joint becomes involved in a sequence of pathological events, including ligament and tendon damage, cartilage destruction, disk herniation, tissue inflammation, etc. The hydraulic conductivity can be broken by temporary or permanent muscle blockade, metabolic processes, or by a combination of both factors.

When tendons pull the periosteum away from the bone, the bone activates the remodeling of its outer surface. The process is called "subperiosteal apposition" (Gray and Lewis 1918). The bone gradually increases in diameter and mass. The growing bone requires a greater blood supply, and more space is needed for the growing bone's marrow. This triggers a mechanism of bone resorption on its inner surface, which forms the marrow canal. While muscle activity is regularly increasing, the periosteum grows, and its growth proceeds with the growth of the bone. Since the bone growth is a consequence of the periosteum's action, it occurs with a certain lag relative to periosteum growth. It is possible to imagine a situation when due to an abrupt interruption in physical activity, the periosteum development stops before the bone's development stops. If this is the case, the growing bone would meet extra tightness from the surrounding periosteum shell. This extra tightness can disrupt the hydraulic conductivity in the tiny space between the periosteum and bone, triggering a negative chain of events.

Decreased hydraulic conductivity between synovial capsules may lead to their hydraulic isolation, meaning that they have to withstand the same loads but without their hydraulic net distribution of pressures.

The limitation of joint articulation will be a logical protective mechanism. However, limited articulation in the joint leads to overloading smaller areas of the cartilage surfaces, and consequently to irreparable damage to the cartilage, which is associated with pain. Pain contributes to a more limited range of motion in joints and to an overall decrease in motor activities. Areas of the joint heads without frequent and regular rolling become filled with connective tissues and osseo-like tissues. Swelling in joints follows, and the liquid captured inside the joint's capsule applies painful pressure. Arthritic symptoms are on their way.

1.5
Future Verification or the Gap Junction Scenario

Focused research needs to be done to morphologically verify the "floating skeleton" concept presented in these pages, since it would be very hard to observe synovial fluid canals along the long bones in vivo. In vitro, these hydraulic structures are probably too fragile to be easily conserved and it would be a challenge to investigate them in cadaver studies.

At the same time, if the hydraulic net does exist, why is the hydraulic connection between any two synovial joints so fragile? In other words, why does the connectivity depend on so tight an attachment of the periosteal layer to the outer surface of the bone?

Let us consider this question from a different angle. Suppose that the hydraulic connection is provided by a loose periosteum or by definite canals like blood vessels. That would immediately require additional means for preventing the synovial fluid in upper joints from moving downward under gravity. In contrast, what we see in an actual normal joint is a fine balance between two dynamic processes. The first process keeps the amount of synovial liquid inside the joint capsule almost constant, and seals it, preventing it from leaking out by tightening the ligaments and periosteum around the epiphyses of the bones forming the joint. The other process must allow a certain amount of synovial liquid to penetrate a tiny canal between the periosteum and the outer surface of the bone's diaphysis along the enthesis.

A possible structure for facilitating the hydraulic connectivity between the synovial joints through the periosteum could be a system of *gap junctions*. A gap junction consists of intercellular channels that provide aqueous continuity between adjacent cells, thus allowing the diffusion of small molecules and ions from cell to cell (Grimston et al. 2008). For example, the gap junctions that form the synapses between neurons providing electrical link is 4 nm wide (1 nm = 10^{-9} m). The gap junction in a synapse for chemical conductive link is 20–40 nm wide. In general, space for hydraulic conductivity via the gap junctions can be offered for molecules whose mass is not greater than 1,000 Da[3] (Kumar and Gilula 1996).

While the composition of synovial liquid is very complex, its main element is water (Lipowitz 1985). A water molecule is 18.01 Da[4] in mass and about 0.2 nm in size. So, even a 1 nm gap between the layers would be sufficient for maintaining hydraulic connectivity in the net. Since the water molecule's mass is about 50 times less than the 1,000 Da threshold for passing the gap junction, a morphological possibility exists of a passage of the synovial liquid through a space between the synovial capsule and the periosteal shell at the level of epiphysis.

With the gap junction scenario, new methods have to be developed for visualizing this structure, since the current method of choice used in investigating orthopedic objects, magnetic resonance imaging (MRI), may not be adequate for the task. MRI distinguishes

---

[3] 1 Da = 1 g/mol
[4] "Atomic Weights and Isotopic Compositions for All Elements," National Institute of Standards and Technology (NIST), 2007

different soft tissues like ligaments, tendons, and muscles in addition to detecting bone tissues like X-rays. The techniques of MRI are based on capturing the spatial distribution of protons passing through live tissues in the external magnetic and radio frequency fields. The magnetic field aligns the magnetic magnetization of hydrogen atoms of water in the body. The radio frequency fields alter the alignment of this magnetization, causing the hydrogen nuclei to produce a rotating magnetic field detectable by the scanner. The signal is an input for a computerized system that reconstructs the image from the object's projections (Novelline and Squire 1997).

An example of effective reconstruction by MRI of the ankle joint (Li et al. 2008) is shown in Fig. 1.3a.

The reason why MRI may not conclusively detect the distribution of synovial liquid under the periosteum is that the quality of the MRI images results from a long process of "teaching" the computerized recognition system. This process requires the scientist and programmer to establish a one-to-one correspondence between the raw signal and the tissues' morphological characteristics. That can be illustrated by comparing the quality of the first published MRI of a human wrist in 1977 (Fig. 1.13) (Hinshaw, Bottomley et al. 1977) with the MRI in Fig 1.3a. While a vast improvement in quality and resolution in the recent image is apparent, it might be not sufficient yet to detect and analyze the hydraulic connection between joints' capsules.

Another issue in interpretation of the MRI and other indirect imaging technologies is that the precise correspondence to the biological substances is based mainly on cadaver studies. Due to the postulated fragility of the skeletal hydraulic net, cadaver studies may not be adequate for verifying the floating skeleton concept.

A possible approach to directly verify the floating skeleton concept could be a new technique developed by Dunkin and colleagues (Dankin et al. 2005) involving local activation of a molecular fluorescent probe (LAMP). The technique was developed for investigating gap junction channels in intact living cells using a new class of photo-activatible fluorophores (Spray 2005).

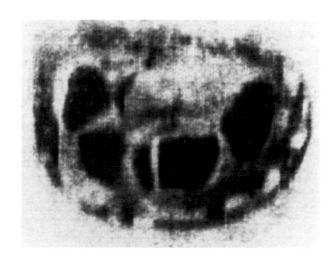

Fig. 1.13 The first published MRI of a human wrist (Adapted from (Hinshaw et al. 1977) with permission from Macmillan Publishers Ltd.)

A mechanism of joint effusion via membrane has been actively investigated (Hopkins, Ingersoll et al. 2001; Palmieri-Smith, Kreinbrink et al. 2007). However, the process of the synovial liquid's spreading along the diaphysis is only hypothesized at this moment. Nevertheless, we believe that there is a strong rationale for considering this process in the biomechanics of protecting the skeleton in anticipation that the experimental verification will be found later on.

1.6
A Common Basis for Therapeutic Procedures

The floating skeleton concept suggests that, at their root, successful therapeutic procedures aim to promote and sustain hydraulic conductivity between joints. While superficially different, procedures such as yoga, proprioceptive neuromuscular facilitation (Knott and Voss 1968), myofascial therapy (Travell and Simons 1983), the savasana principle (Pitkin 1991), and manipulative techniques such as massage and chiropractic therapy (Palmer 1910; Brunarski 1984; Cramer et al. 2006), all have a common aim.

On the foundation of Emanuel Swedenborg's theories introduced in the mid-eighteenth century (Swedenborg 1882; Jordan 2009), William Sutherland developed cranial osteopathy (Upledger and Vredevoogd 1983). The osteopathic physician induces micro articular mobility of the cranial bones, targeting the dura mater that covers the brain. Since the dural membranes are positioned under the skull, and the skull has an outer periosteum (*pericarnium*) and an inner periosteum (*endocranium*), the relative movements of the cranial bones affect and hopefully restore the hydraulic conductivity between the skull and the spine. Even in case of success, specialists in their respective fields are often uncertain about the mechanism by which the technique applied to a patient leads to improvement. For example, in a recent comparative study on treatment of chronic neck pain, two groups of patients treated with chiropractics and physical exercises showed statistically significant improvement. However, no difference was found between the groups (Murphy et al. 2010).

As we postulate here, therapies are as successful as the degree to which they are able to restore hydraulic conductivity of the skeleton's elastic shell.

When the skeletal muscle moves the limb during exercise, it simultaneously pulls away the periosteum in the enthesis zone. This action naturally pumps liquid through the space between the periosteum and the bone, which, according to our hypothesis, helps maintain the hydraulic connection between joints. Once the hydraulic connection is complete, the skeleton can withhold the required loads and be responsive to the associated muscles' actions, pumping the needed amount of liquid into the hydraulic net.

If the hydraulic net is broken, however, those movements which used to be encouraged by the body may become harmful. In such a case the restoration of the hydraulic connection between the joints may require a different approach than traditional therapeutic procedures. I call this approach sanomechanics. Sanomechanics focuses on creating favorable conditions for the distribution of synovial liquid via capillarity and osmosis. These are the conditions I will describe in the next chapters.

1.7
First Experimental Evidence of the Hydraulic Connection Between Joints

In order for relative rolling to be possible during articulation, as in flexion and extension, the contacting surfaces in a joint are not congruent. Consequently, when the joint's angle changes, the space between the contacting surfaces changes as well, causing a change in pressure inside the synovial capsule. If a hydraulic connection between joints exists, as the concept of the floating skeleton postulates, pressure changes in one joint should affect the pressure in other joints' capsules.

There are several reports on the investigations of the pressure–angle relations in a single joint (Levick 1979; Knight and Levick 1985; McDonald and Levick 1995; Gardner et al. 1998; van Valburg et al. 2000; Lee et al. 2008). Knight and Levick conducted simultaneous measurements in two opposite knee joints with one joint flexed at different angles and the other joint in an extended position as a control (Knight and Levick 1982). The authors reported that pressure was much greater in the flexed joint than in the control joint, but they did not indicate whether the pressure in the control joint remained the same or was changing in response to the flexions in the driving joint.

Since the latter question is essential for experimental verification of the hydraulic connection between joints, a pilot study was organized as a part of a closely related project.[5] A protocol for the study was developed, submitted to, and approved by the IACUC[6] of the Pine Acre Rabbitry Farm, a certified animal facility in Norton, MA. The pressures in two joints were simultaneously measured, where one of the joints was articulated, while the second remained motionless. The experiment was performed on two New Zealand rabbits.

Through one cannula inserted in the knee capsule, and another cannula inserted in the ankle capsule, the pressures in both capsules were simultaneously measured with two independent pressure transducer systems (Deltatran® IV[7]). The synovial fluid hydrostatic pressure was recorded when either the ankle or knee joint was fixed and the other joint was a driver (flexed and extended ten times with two articulations per second).

During the course of the tests, the pressure in the articulating joint was increasing two to four times on average, which was in accord with published data (Yen et al. 2009). The new result was that the pressure in the motionless joint was also increasing, and at a similar rate. The rise in pressure in the motionless joint generated by the increased pressure in the articulated joint should be seen as an indication of the hydraulic conductivity between the joints, where the excessive pressure can be transmitted without flow of fluid. A possibility still exists that tendons acting on both the ankle and knee joints may contribute to the changes in pressure of the fixed joint. As the study is ongoing, and a full report will only be published upon its completion, I wanted to inform the readers here about this first direct experimental argument in support of the floating skeleton concept.

[5]NIH Grant R44HD057492: Manufacturing technology for skin integrated composite prosthetic pylon
[6]Institutional Animal Care and Use Committee
[7]Utah Medical Products, Inc., Midvale, UT 84047

References

Alexander R (1987) Bending of cylindrical animals with helical fibres in their skin or cuticle. J Theor Biol 124:97–110

Alexander RM (1968) Animal mechanics. Sidgwick & Jackson, London

Anderson AE, Ellis BJ et al (2008) Validation of finite element predictions of cartilage contact pressure in the human hip joint. J Biomech Eng 130(5):051008

Barra JG, Crottogini AJ et al (2004) Contribution of myocardium hydraulic skeleton to left ventricular wall interaction and synergy in dogs. Am J Physiol Heart Circ Physiol 287(2):H896–H904

Bartelink DL (1957) The role of abdominal pressure in relieving the pressure on the lumbar intervertebral discs. J Bone Joint Surg Br 39-B(4):718–725

Batchelor GK (1967) An introduction to fluid dynamics. Cambridge University Press, Cambridge

Benjamin M, McGonagle D (2001) The anatomical basis for disease localisation in seronegative spondyloarthropathy at entheses and related sites. J Anat 199(Pt 5):503–526

Benjamin M, McGonagle D (2009) Entheses: tendon and ligament attachment sites. Scand J Med Sci Sports 19(4):520–527

Borelli GA (1680) De Motu Animalium. Princeton University Press, Princeton

Brunarski D (1984) Clinical trials of spinal manipulation: a critical appraisal and review of the literature. J Manipulative Physiol Ther 7(4):243–249

Casey TM (1991) Energetics of caterpillar locomotion: biomechanical constraints of a hydraulic skeleton. Science 252(5002):112–114

Cramer G, Budgell B et al (2006) "Basic science research related to chiropractic spinal adjusting: the state of the art and recommendations revisited." J Manipulative Physiol Ther 29(9): 726–761

Dankin K, Zhao Y et al (2005) LAMP, a new imaging assay of gap junctional communication unveils that Ca^{2+} influx inhibits cell coupling. Nat Methods 2:55–62

Elftman H (1938) The measurement of the external force in walking. Science 88:152–153

Falkovich G, Weinberg A et al (2005) Surface tension: floater clustering in a standing wave. Nature 435(7045):1045–1046

Fick JM, Thambyah A et al (2010) Articular cartilage compression: how microstructural response influences pore pressure in relation to matrix health. Connect Tissue Res 51(2):132–149

Foolen J, van Donkelaar C et al (2008) Collagen orientation in periosteum and perichondrium is aligned with preferential directions of tissue growth. J Orthop Res 26(9):1263–1268

Gardner TN, Evans M, Simpson H, Kenwright J (1998) Force-displacement behaviour of biological tissue during distraction osteogenesis. Med Eng Phys 20(9):708–715

Granata KP, Marras WS et al (1997) Biomechanical assessment of lifting dynamics, muscle activity and spinal loads while using three different styles of lifting belt. Clin Biomech (Bristol Avon) 12(2):107–115

Gray H, Lewis WH (1918) Anatomy of the human body. Lea & Febiger, Philadelphia, Bartleby. com, 2000. www.bartleby.com/1-7/

Greene GW, Zappone B, Zhao B, Soderman O, Topgaard D, Rata G, Israelachvili JN (2008) Changes in pore morphology and fluid transport in compressed articular cartilage and the implications for joint lubrication. Biomaterials. 29(33):4455–4462

Grimston SK, Brodt MD et al (2008) Attenuated response to in vivo mechanical loading in mice with conditional osteoblast ablation of the connexin43 gene (Gja1). J Bone Miner Res 23(6):879–886

Grotberg J, Jensen O (2004) Biofluid mechanics in flexible tube. Annu Rev Fluid Mech 36:121–147

Hinshaw WS, Bottomley PA et al (1977) Radiographic thin-section image of the human wrist by nuclear magnetic resonance. Nature 270(5639):722–723

Hodge WA, Fijan RS et al (1986) Contact pressures in the human hip joint measured in vivo. Proc Natl Acad Sci USA 83(9):2879–2883

Hopkins JT, Ingersoll CD et al (2001) Effect of knee joint effusion on quadriceps and soleus motoneuron pool excitability. Med Sci Sports Exerc 33(1):123–126

Jordan T (2009) Swedenborg's influence on Sutherland's 'Primary Respiratory Mechanism' model in cranial osteopathy. International Journal of Osteopathic Medicine 12(3): 100–105

Knight AD, Levick JR (1982) Pressure-volume relationships above and below atmospheric pressure in the synovial cavity of the rabbit knee. J Physiol 328:403–420

Knight AD, Levick JR (1985) Effect of fluid pressure on the hydraulic conductance of interstitium and fenestrated endothelium in the rabbit knee. J Physiol 360:311–332

Knott M, Voss DE (1968) Proprioceptive neuromuscular facilitation: patterns and techniques. Hoeber Medical Division, New York

Koehl M, Quillin K et al (2000) Mechanical design of fiber-wound hydraulic skeletons: the stiffening and straightening of embryonic notochords. Am Zool 40:28–41

Kumar NM, Gilula NB (1996) The gap junction communication channel. Cell 84(3):381–388

Lee KJ, Lee HD, Chung SG (2008) Real-time pressure monitoring of intraarticular hydraulic distension for painful stiff shoulders. J Orthop Res 26(7):965–970

Leroy Y, Cathey S, et al (2009) Mucolipidosis II. In: Pagon RA, Bird TC, Dolan CR, Stephens K (eds) GeneReviews: http://www.ncbi.nlm.nih.gov/books/NBK1828/

Levick JR (1979) An investigation into the validity of subatmospheric pressure recordings from synovial fluid and their dependence on joint angle. J Physiol 289:55–67

Li G, Wan L et al (2008) Determination of real-time in-vivo cartilage contact deformation in the ankle joint. J Biomech 41(1):128 136

Lipowitz AJ (1985) Synovial fluid. In: Newton C, Nunamaker D (eds) Textbook of small animal orthopaedics. Lippincott Williams & Wilkins, Ithaca

Lunkenheimer PP, Ising H (1974) The hydraulic skeleton of the heart. A working hypothesis on the mechanism of ventricle unfolding. Zentralbl Veterinärmed A 21(5):365–378

McDonald JN, Levick JR (1995) Effect of intra-articular hyaluronan on pressure-flow relation across synovium in anaesthetized rabbits. J Physiol 485(Pt 1):179–193

Michael JA, Sircar S (2010) Fundamentals of medical physiology. Thieme, New York

Milz S, Boszczyk BM et al (2005) The enthesis. Physiological morphology, molecular composition and pathoanatomical alterations. Orthopade 34(6):526–532

Murphy B, Taylor HH et al (2010) The effect of spinal manipulation on the efficacy of a rehabilitation protocol for patients with chronic neck pain: a pilot study. J Manipulative Physiol Ther 33(3):168–177

Nordin M, Kahanovitz N et al (1987) Normal trunk muscle strength and endurance in women and the effect of exercises and electrical stimulation. Part 1: normal endurance and trunk muscle strength in 101 women. Spine 12(2):105–111

Novelline RA, Squire LF (1997) Squire's fundamentals of radiology. Harvard University Press, Cambridge

Palmieri-Smith RM, Kreinbrink J et al (2007) Quadriceps inhibition induced by an experimental knee joint effusion affects knee joint mechanics during a single-legged drop landing. Am J Sports Med 35(8):1269–1275

Palmer DD (1910) The Chiropractor's Adjuster: A Textbook of the Science, Art, and Philosophy of Chiropractic for Students and Practitioners. Portland, OR, Portland Printing House

Perry J (1992) Gait analysis: normal and pathological function. Slack, Inc., Thorofare

Pitkin M (1991) A new biomechanical technique for increasing of joint flexibility with a focus on back pain prevention. In: Proceedings of the XIII international congress of biomechanics, the University of Western Australia, Australia, 9–13 Dec 1991, pp 243–244

Pitkin M (1993) Floating skeleton concept to explain causes of injuries in spine and success of any therapeutic procedure. In: Proceedings of the XIV international conference ISB, Paris, France, 1993, pp 1052–1053

Pitkin MR (2010) Biomechanics of lower limb prosthetics. Springer, New York

Rawls ES (1966) A handbook of yoga for modern living. Parker Publication Co., West Nyack

Rufai A, Ralphs JR et al (1996) Ultrastructure of fibrocartilages at the insertion of the rat Achilles tendon. J Anat 189(Pt 1):185–191

Sack L, Cowan PD et al (2003) The "hydrology" of leaves: co-ordination of structure and function in temperate woody species. Plant Cell Environ 26(26):1343–1356

Schneidman E, Bialek W et al (2003) Synergy, redundancy, and independence in population codes. J Neurosci 23(37):11539–11553

Simon SR (2004) Quantification of human motion: gait analysis-benefits and limitations to its application to clinical problems. J Biomech 37(12):1869–1880

Spray D (2005) Illuminating gap junctions. Nat Methods 2:12–14

Squier CA, Ghoneim S et al (1990) Ultrastructure of the periosteum from membrane bone. J Anat 171:233–239

Sutherland W (1998) Contributions of thought: collected writings of William Garner Sutherland, DO. 2nd ed. Portland OR, Rudra Press

Swedenborg E (1882) The brain, considered anatomically, physiologically and philosophically. London, James Speirs

Thompson JW, Sorvig K (2008) Sustainable landscape construction: a guide to green building outdoors. Island Press, Washington

Travell JG, Simons DG (1983) Myofascial pain and dysfunction: the trigger point manual. Williams & Wilkins, Baltimore

Tyree MT, Frank EW (1992) The hydraulic architecture of trees and other woody plants. New Phytol 119(3):345–360

Upledger JE, Vredevoogd JD (1983) Craniosacral therapy. Eastland Press, Chicago

van Dijk JH (1979) A theory on the control of arbitrary movements. Biol Cybern 32(4):187–199

van Valburg AA, van Roermund PM, Marijnissen AC, Wenting MJ, Verbout AJ, Lafeber FP, Bijlsma JW (2000) Joint distraction in treatment of osteoarthritis (II): effects on cartilage in a canine model. Osteoarthritis Cartilage 8(1):1–8

Winter DA (1979) Biomechanics of human movement. John Wiley & Sons, Inc., New York

Winter DA (1991) The biomechanics and motor control of human gait: normal, elderly and pathological. University of Waterloo Press, Ontario

Yen CH, Leung HB, Tse PY (2009) Effects of hip joint position and intra-capsular volume on hip joint intra-capsular pressure: a human cadaveric model. J Orthop Surg Res 4:8

Sanomechanics

2

2.1
Sanomechanical Approach to Exercises

The systems of perfecting body and mind through systematic exercises usually try to unite the physical aspects of the routine with a philosophical background. Sanomechanics as a system does the same. What distinguishes sanomechanics from other systems is its foundation in the floating skeleton concept. Relying on this new, biomechanically justified concept, sanomechanics consists of the corresponding technique, autosuggestion and criterion of correctness of performance. The structure of the sanomechanical approach to exercise is schematically depicted in Fig. 2.1 (where the "biomechanical concept" was presented and discussed in Chap. 1). The conceptual autosuggestion, technique, and criterion of correctness of performance, their biomechanical justification will be discussed below.

2.2
Conceptual Autosuggestion

2.2.1
Biomechanics of Visualization and Anticipation

Visualization is a way of seeing beyond what the eyes see. An image either appears when we consciously suggest it to our mind, or uncontrollably, as in dreams. Visualization is the bridge between our conscious and subconscious, and a tool for their interaction. Just as any tool, it can be useful if used properly, or useless and harmful otherwise. The spectrum of focused applications of visualization is very wide, ranging from athletes who hope to improve their performance to autogenic training and religious mysticism.

People have harnessed the power of visualization through meditation for thousands of years. Only in the past decades have neurological advances permitted us to begin to understand the link between mental visualization and the attendant physiological responses. Visualization, when applied to biomechanics, would require a person to select an image from a mental "library" of images, and guided by it, to coordinate his or her body segment's movements.

M.R. Pitkin, *Biomechanics for Life*, 25
DOI: 10.1007/978-3-642-17177-2_2, © Springer-Verlag Berlin Heidelberg 2011

Fig. 2.1 Structure of the
method of sanomechanics

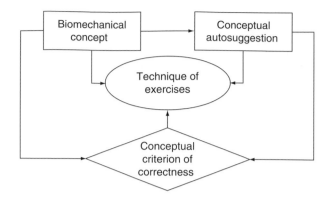

The physiological mechanism called *anticipation* is a generalization of visualization. It is the brain's ability to predict movements and prepare the body for its tasks. Unlike visualization, anticipation does not require a definite image. It is a preplan for a goal-oriented movement in response to a visual or verbal stimulus, or for a movement generated by reflex. An example is the goal of maintaining balance while walking. The goal is a achieved with a preplan for how to respond to external disturbances, like a patch of ice on the sidewalk, or your name yelled out across the street. With anticipation, the body is aware of the imminent task, and reacts faster than when the task comes abruptly. Naturally, the body's reaction is safer when it is prepared (Houck et al. 2006).

The human skeleton has more than 200 movable joints. The joints have one, two or three degrees of freedom, and almost each degree of freedom can be operated independently. Controlling body movements with both speed and precision in order to reach purposeful outcomes is therefore a great challenge. The breakthrough explanation of how the body meets this challenge was proposed by Nikolai Bernstein (Бернштейн 1927, 1947; Bernstein 1967), who suggested that certain degrees of freedom can be controlled together by one parameter synergistically.[1] According to the theory, goal-oriented actions of the body are organized through hierarchical top-down control, where the bottom levels are devoted to automatic and instinctual movements, freeing the higher levels to respond to new and unexpected tasks.

When a person is standing and is told to raise his hand, his conditions of balance change, and without compensatory action, the innocent arm raise will jeopardize his balance and safety. The system of posture control prevents him from falling. The posture control directs synchronous movements of body segments, adjusting to the movement of the arm automatically. An analysis detected a delay (latent period) of 130–140 ms (1 ms = 10^{-3} sec) between the time when a subject was given the command to raise his hand and the beginning of movements (Belen'kii et al. 1967). The latent period depends on the nature of the task that the body performs. If the task is expected, the latent period is shorter, and if the task is an unexpected perturbation, the latent period is longer. When the task is preplanned,

---

[1]*Synergy* from Greek *syn-ergos* (working together)

the control system can use the more standard programs of synergistic movements in the required degrees of freedom of the body. When the task is unplanned, it takes additional time to adjust the standard programs adequately.

The latent period of muscle response is also age dependent, and increases with age (Inglin and Woollacott 1988), especially for unexpected perturbations. To maintain safety, a compensatory strategy of generalized stiffening through co-contraction may be developed, as suggested by Maki (1993). The body's stiffening in the elderly corresponds to the process of a decrease in the range of motion (flexibility) in joints (Nigg and Skleryk 1988; Bassey et al. 1989).

The complexity of controlling movements in multiple degrees of freedom can be appreciated if we, following the studies conducted by Nikolai Bernstein in 1930 (Bernstein 1930), look at how a pianist presses the piano key. We began by positioning the index finger on an A key in a "regular" fashion, as shown in Fig. 2.2. The pianist was asked to press the same key with different configurations of the arm (Fig. 2.3), without changing the position of the torso. In this setting, the distance between the shoulder joint and the piano key remained unchanged. The shoulder joint has three degrees of freedom; the elbow joint has one; the

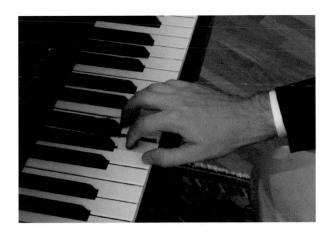

Fig. 2.2 Positioning of the index finger on the piano key "Λ" with standard angulations in its phalanges, as well as in the wrist, elbow, and shoulder joints

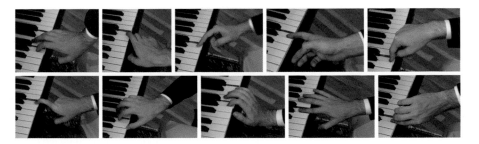

Fig. 2.3 The same end positioning of the index finger on the "A" key (as shown at the top left), but with different angulations in the joints of the arm

wrist, three; the finger, three. So the tip of the finger is an end point of a poly-linker with ten degrees of freedom. Figure 2.3 shows ten configurations of the arm, representing a tiny fraction of the total number of possible configurations that solve the experiment's task.

Now, let us turn to the reality of playing a piece of music, when the fingers have to press many keys in a predetermined time sequence (tempo/rhythm). We immediately see a dramatic reduction of the number of possible configurations of the arm. Moreover, even if the piece is played by different musicians, their respective patterns of arm movements are remarkably similar to each other's, with minor individual differences. The phenomenon of such a stable pattern of pre-trained movements can be explained by the concept of joint synergies as well.

The development of synergies allows the motion of many segments to be organized and controlled by a single parameter. If we try to imagine how many degrees of freedom there are in internal organs, vessels, and soft tissues, we realize that control over the motion of body segments is just the tip of the iceberg. In this book, we will work towards achieving the goal of restoring and activating the hydraulic net around our skeleton. This task also requires precise control over the performance of all components of the net. To provide this control, we need to inform the body of what is anticipated in the course of exercising according to the new *floating skeleton* concept. The best way to do this is to develop a specific autosuggestion, and to use it during exercise sessions.

2.2.2
Autosuggestion

In a sense, autosuggestion is a goal-oriented anticipation of a body's reaction to a task. Autosuggestion as a healing factor was introduced by Emile Coué (Coué 1923), who has written about its closeness to meditation. He also stressed that it was only realistic outcomes – not miracles – that could be expected.

The second milestone in broadly introducing therapeutic autosuggestions to the masses was the development of *autogenic training* by Schultz in 1932 (Luthe and Schultz 1969). The method includes a special relaxation technique designed to increase the acceptance of autosuggestion by the body and mind (suggestibility). Dr. Schultz found that natural suggestibility reaches its maximal level in the morning during the transition from sleep to wakefulness.

The next step in making autogenic therapy a successful methodology was made by Sonya Lyubinskaya, who formulated a rule called the "right to autosuggestion" (Lyubinskaya 1970). A person must "earn" the right to practice autosuggestion by taking adequate preparatory measures, i.e., meeting certain preconditions. For example, if a person wishes to restore his or her energy, the autosuggestion "I feel more energetic and less tired" will work only if the person is genuinely willing to improve his lifestyle, eating habits, etc. The autosuggestion "I will earn a high score on my exam" is useful only after the person has dutifully attended lecture and read his notes.

For all sanomechanical exercises, we will invoke the image of a skeleton, with synovial liquid filling the space between the bones' surfaces and the periosteum. The image is based on the concept of the floating skeleton (Chap. 1) and will be used to develop the sanomechanical autosuggestion. We must visualize this image; in combination with the *criterion of correctness of the exercise* to be discussed below, it will provide us with the right to sanomechanical auto suggestion: "My skeleton in totally immersed in synovial fluid."

2.3
Criterion of Correctness of the Exercise

2.3.1
Level of Sensation

It is good to know, before embarking on an exercise, how we will control its duration, associated loads, and ranges of motion. We need a criterion or criteria of correctness for our exercises, which can minimize the risks and maximize the positive effects of the exercises.

In sanomechanical exercises, I suggest that a *hedonic[2] criterion*, based on the pleasurable signal coming from the involved zones of the body, be used to evaluate the exercise's correctness. The hedonic criterion loosely finds its philosophical grandfather in the *pleasure principle* proposed by Sigmund Freud with his hierarchy of the psyche: *id–ego–super ego*.

In the *pleasure principle*, Freud ascribed the motivating and rewarding signals of pleasure to a person's *id* lying at the bottom of the psyche's hierarchy. In Freud's theory, the person's *ego* and *super ego* have to suppress the *id's* desire of perpetually remaining in the pleasure zone, in order to set up and solve the tasks of higher importance. The requests for pleasure from the *id* are constrained by Freud's *reality principle,* which separates the "good" requests from the "bad" according to standards meaningful for the person.

For the purpose of *sanomechanical* theory, let us borrow Freud's terminology, and speak of the physical body's or skeleton's unconscious requests as those coming from the id. These requests may be for pleasure, or for the avoidance of pain. These signals can also be suppressed by reality. For example, a surgeon will continue a procedure until its completion, even if his feet feel pain for having stood for a long time. Or, one might not stretch in the boardroom, no matter how pleasurable the stretch, because it would contradict the code of social conduct.

When we reach a point of unhappiness with our health, we may realize by looking back that in the past we did not follow and did not respect some legitimate requests from the body. So, to stop or at least to slow down our health's decline let us elevate the meaning of the pleasure signal from the skeleton by accepting its importance through the *super ego*. It will give us a hedonic criterion of correctness of our actions during exercising. From now on, according to the criterion, let us nourish the pleasure signal from the skeleton, rather than suppress it. Compared to many of the *id*'s other pleasure requests like those associated with hunger or sexuality, the requests from our skeleton, if met, do not have potential negative side effects. As to the positive consequences, they were presented and discussed in Chap. 1 and will be made more evident in Chap. 5.

---

[2]The term *hedonic* means "related to pleasure" from the Greek *hēdonē*, pleasure

Each relative position of body segments produces one of three basic types of signals to the brain: zero/neutral, pleasure, and pain. When you read a book – for example, when you read this page – your head's position is determined by what is convenient for your eyes. At the same time, this position is probably comfortable enough for your neck. If it is comfortable indeed, you may say that the neck generates a zero/neutral signal. If the position generates pain then you, like everyone else, will (or should) alter it in an attempt to eliminate or minimize the pain. That unconscious change in neck position will be an action generated by your *id*. If your *ego* or *super ego* insists on the critical importance of continuing the reading uninterrupted, you will comply, leaving the pain signal unaddressed at least for a while. If suppressing or ignoring the pain signal becomes a pattern, it may cause *osteochondritis*,[3] and the first and most straightforward recommendation from your doctor would be to avoid the painful position of the neck during reading. To use Freud's terminology, the recommendation is to teach your *super ego* not to suppress the pain signal from the *id*.

A fundamental fact is that between the neutral and painful zones there is an interval that gives a sense of pleasure. We need to examine the nature of the pleasure signal from our joints in order to understand the purpose and the aim of such encouragement.

The signals entering the brain and informing it about the situation at the periphery are called *afferent* signals, whereas the brain sends *efferent* signals as commands back to the periphery. Usually, routine locomotion and familiar movements are organized in such a way as to reduce the inflow of signals, and this tendency is called the *principle of minimization of afferent information.* Those movements which are new and require learning, like new professional or athletic techniques, generate an influx of afferent information, which is diminished once the movements become more automatic.

Let us ask ourselves: why, in the course of an automatic routine's development, does the body not try to increase the inflow of pleasure signals, but organizes the motions to generate a lesser and lesser volume of afferent signals? To find the answer we need to go beyond biomechanics and to enter the philosophy of a human life's purpose. In a broad sense, the purpose is to modify the environment. The purpose is ambitious indeed and requires guidance from the *super ego*, not the *id*. Cyclic routines have to use a small part of the brain's controlling capacity, leaving its major power for solving extraordinary tasks in the quickly changing and dangerous world surrounding us.

Generally, pleasure is the signal of a useful stimulus, and pain is a signal of danger. Usefulness or danger in maintaining homeostasis and in achieving higher human aims is judged by the peripheral and central nervous system. A hedonic hierarchy is thereby established, with positive and negative values of stimuli, where the higher levels have supremacy over the lower levels, and where physiological stimuli are mixed and bound with the psychological. Positive values relate to pleasure (Cabanac 1979) and negative values relate to displeasure (Hoffman et al. 2008). Over a lifetime, the stimuli may change their position in the hierarchy, thereby directly or indirectly affecting our motivations and behavior. They may change their position several times within a day, like the desire to eat (appetite), which goes up in the hierarchy when we are hungry and goes down as we consume enough

---

[3]Inflammation of bone and cartilage

food. An abrupt jump to the highest priority of a stimulus may occur any time if related to protecting the body's integrity, such as when we are burned. The changes in priorities are described by Sigmund Freud as the constant conflict of the *reality principle* and the *pleasure principle* (Freud 1929). We may say that a person establishes for himself/herself and chooses to follow the *hedonic criterion* as result of a victory of Freud's *pleasure principle* over the *reality principle*. It is a victory driven by the person's *id*, but proclaimed and confirmed by the person's *ego* and *super ego*.

We already spoke about positioning the head while reading. Once we feel that the reading is important, either for giving us intellectual pleasure or meeting professional needs, we may and we almost certainly do automatically suppress the demand from the neck to find a position in which the sensation of pleasure would be maximized. We prefer reading with an indifferent afferent signal from the neck. It is convenient indeed, since it allows us to concentrate on the contents of the reading material in front of us, instead of sharing our attention with analyzing the neck's well-being. The reality principle assigns higher priority to reading and lower priority to the neck's pleasure. The reward comes or is anticipated to come from the sphere of psychology rather than the body's physiology.

The situation may change if a negative hedonic signal (pain) tells us that our neck is in trouble. If the signal is tolerable, we may choose not to react and continue what we were doing before. However, if the pain persists, its priority in the hedonic hierarchy goes up, until it exceeds that of reading. At this point, we have to address the pain somehow. For instance, we may change the neck's position or massage it. We may simply stop reading. In worse scenarios, we opt for treatment. However, the best way to address the situation would be to do a couple of exercises, to be described soon.

2.3.2
Pleasure Signal from Joints and from Muscles

Pain and pleasure – these are the two most informative "words" in the language through which the body and the mind communicate. These two "words" come from various locations in the body, and with different levels of intensity and duration. Sometimes, the message is clear, but most of the time, it has to be decoded in order to better understand it and to respond. Such decoding may require collecting and analyzing data from medical tests. All organs and systems in the body use this language directly or indirectly. The sense of pleasure encourages us toward certain actions and rewards us for doing certain things, while pain serves as a discouraging warning or punishment for something.

Below is a portrait of muscular pleasure presented by Dr. Thomas Brown in his *Lectures on the Philosophy of the Mind* (Brown 1822).

> Muscular pleasure of alacrity and action forms so great a part of the delight of the young of every species of living beings and is felt, though in a less degree, at every period of life …. that doubles to every one the delight of exercise by sweetening the repose to which it leads, and thus making it indirectly, as well as directly, a source of enjoyment.

In response to muscle exercises, the body produces dopamine, which contributes to the pleasure sensation (Arakawa 2002; Foley and Fleshner 2008). Activation of muscles attached to the bones periodically pulls the periosteum away from the bone surfaces and in this way improves the hydraulic connectivity of the joints. Therefore, the chemical mechanism of encouragement of the muscle workout and development indirectly rewards the restoration of the skeleton's hydraulic net. That chemical mechanism may mask a direct signal of pleasure from the articulation in a particular joint. We therefore need to learn how to listen to that voice with our full attention, and respectfully follow its humble requests, giving them higher priority.

Based on the floating skeleton concept, we assume that the pleasure signal from the joints is an encouragement for creating and maintaining conditions for the restoration of the hydraulic net of all synovial joints. At the same time, it may coincide with the encouragement for activity in muscles, and for a regenerative effect in the joint cartilages as the mobility in joints increases (Salter 1994).

2.3.3
Duration of Keeping a Position

Understanding and addressing the body's pleasure signal is easy and enjoyable. When I bend my torso forward, trying to touch the floor with my fingers, I hold my position as soon as the encouragement zone is reached, and stay in this position until the pleasure subsides. I don't try anymore, like I did in my younger years, to cross the pleasure threshold and enter the pain zone, in attempts to increase my range of motion.

2.4
Technique of Exercising

The technique of exercising is at the core of sanomechanics. It includes informational and instructional parts for the mind and for the body. We will observe the technique now, since we have already become familiar with conceptual autosuggestion, and with criterion of correctness of performance.

The sanomechanical autosuggestion:

"My skeleton in totally immersed in the synovial fluid" will work to maximize the effectiveness of your exercises because you can now visualize the concept and activate a mechanism of anticipation for optimal selection of synergies.

You are already familiar with the hedonic criterion of correctness of performance and you understand the nature of the feedback that the body generates in response to the current angle in a joint. You know that the sensation of pleasure we find at a certain angle in the joint encourages us to keep that angle and to hold that position until the signal disappears. We know the purpose of this holding in space and time: the joint becomes hydraulically connected to the entire skeletal net.

As any joint sends feedback signals to the nervous system about its well-being, the signal may be neutral, encouraging, or discouraging. A neutral signal conveys that in this zone of the joint's anatomical range of motion, mobility is not restricted. An encouraging/pleasurable signal comes when the amplitude of articulation is extended outside of the neutral zone and it tells us that by holding this angle, we benefit our body. Once articulation continues, the encouraging feedback signal transforms into a discouraging one and very soon becomes a signal of pain.

The structure of mobility zones of a typical joint at the beginning of the sanomechanical series (position 1) is depicted in Fig. 2.4 (replica of Fig. 1.12). It shows zone A_1 where mobility is unrestricted and the sensation feedback is neutral; zones B_1- and B_1+, where the feedback signal becomes encouraging; and zones C_1- and C_1+ with the pain signal. The ranges for zones A, B, and C are very individual and are different not only for the different joints, but for the different degrees of freedom in each of them.

The level of the feedback signal, as a function of the angle in a joint, is schematically depicted in Fig. 2.5, where the joint angle zones correspond to the diagram in Fig. 2.4. In addition to the ranges of zones A, B, and C, the amplitudes of the signals are strictly individual, and may not be symmetrical as shown.

Attributing any position of the joint to a specific zone also depends on how long the joint remains in that zone. For example, if one keeps the head in a neutral position without any pleasant or unpleasant sensation for a long time, a sensation of tiredness and even pain may appear. The sanomechanical technique recognizes that the encouragement/pleasure sensation also diminishes with time.

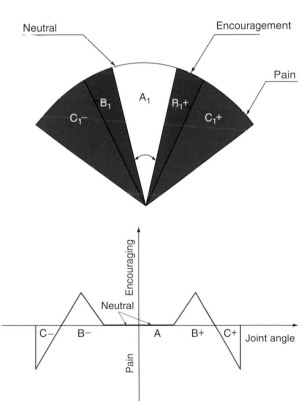

Fig. 2.4 Zones of mobility of a joint in position 1. A_1, unrestricted neutral zone; B_1- and B_1+, encouragement zones; C_1- and C_1+, pain zones

Fig. 2.5 A chart of the feedback sensation the body gets in response to a changing angle in a typical joint. *Blue* – encouraging/ pleasure signal; *red* – discouraging/pain signal. The joint angle zones correspond to the diagram in Fig. 2.4

2.4.1
Cycles of Changing the Joint Angle

- We begin any sanomechanical exercise in the middle of zone A_1, as the initial position 1 (Fig. 2.4) where the sensation is neutral (Fig. 2.5).
- Next, we move within zone A_1, to its border with the zone B_1+, where the sensation is encouraging.
- When we enter zone B_1+ we hold the position, for as long as the encouragement/pleasure feedback is sensed.
- We may carefully move within B_1+, but not enter the zone of pain C_1+.
- Once the encouragement/pleasure signal disappears, we may continue articulation, looking for the next encouragement zone B_2+ in position 2 (Fig. 2.6).
- We stay in zone B_2+ until the encouragement/pleasure signal disappears. That will complete the first cycle of the exercise: transfer from position 1 to position 2.
- We will see that the combined range of motion of zones A_2 and B_2+ in position 2 will be greater than the combined range of motion of zones A_1 and B_1+ in position 1.
- Then, we may go to the next cycles of transfer: from position 2 to position 3, and finally from position 3 to position 4, with position 3 and 4 defined the same way as positions 1 and 2.
- We complete the exercise by returning to position 1, and may repeat it, moving in the other direction.

2.4.2
Example of a Sanomechanical Exercise

Here is a typical sanomechanical exercise. Figure 2.7 (R) depicts three cycles of bending from the neutral position (1) to the right (2,3,4). Figure 2.7 (L) shows the neck bending from the neutral position (1) to the left (2,3,4). All cycles have to be performed very slowly, without any tension.

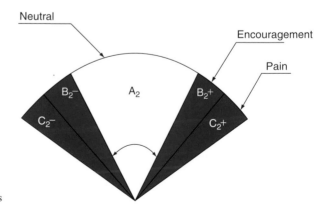

Fig. 2.6 Zones of mobility of a joint in position 2. A_2, new unrestricted neutral zone (compare with Fig. 2.4); B_2- and B_2+, encouragement zones; C_2- and C_2+, pain zones

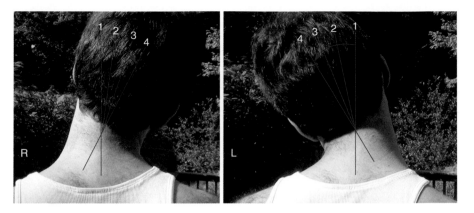

Fig. 2.7 R, bending the neck from the neutral position (1) to the right (2,3,4); L, bending the neck from the neutral position (1) to the left (2,3,4)

- Step 1. Confirm to yourself that the current position (Fig. 2.7 (R,1)) of your neck generates neither a signal of pleasure, nor of displeasure.
- Step 2. Tell yourself:
  - "I am going to lean my head to the right so slowly that a casual observer might not notice it."
  - "I will stop bending and will slowly return back if a sensation of displeasure or pain arises."
  - "I will stop bending when a sensation of pleasure arises, and will stay in that position until the sensation of pleasure disappears. I will then continue to position 2 (Fig. 2.7 (R,2)) or return to the neutral position."
- Step 3. Begin bending your neck as slowly as you instructed yourself and with the end points described in Step 2.
- Step 4. You may do all positions 1,2,3,4, or return back to neutral position 1 based on your feeling.
- Step 5. Repeat Steps 1–4 for bending to the left (Fig. 2.7 (L)).

I hope that the experiments will go well and you will feel some relief in the neck.

2.5
Conclusion

You might feel shy about doing sanomechanical exercises as often as you feel is needed, since other people around might see you, and you are not comfortable with it. You understand that the people around are not comfortable either, watching you in strange postures.

To deal with this feeling you may first recall wether you have ever seen someone running in the street, or stretching, or doing tai chi or yoga in the park or somewhere else? What was your reaction, what did you think about these people, if you thought about them at all?

Most likely you have seen people who were exercising without being self-conscious. Most likely you told yourself: "I would do it also, if I had enough time, appropriate apparel, a place for changing and taking a shower, or if I were younger and slimmer."

Then imagine that someone who is less fit, older, and heavier is watching you exercising and thinks about you as a model to follow. Would not you be willing to help someone who needs your example?

References

Arakawa K (2002) Mild physical exercise may activate the adenosine-dopamine system: a new natriuretic mechanism. Curr Hypertens Rep 4(1):1–2

Bassey EJ, Morgan K et al (1989) Flexibility of the shoulder joint measured as range of abduction in a large representative sample of men and women over 65 years of age. Eur J Appl Physiol Occup Physiol 58(4):353–360

Belen'kii VE, Gurfinkel VS et al (1967) Control elements of voluntary movements. Biofizika 12(1):135–141

Bernstein N (1930) Studies on biodynamics of a piano strike (Rus). Medgiz, Moscow

Bernstein N (1967) The co-ordination and regulation of movements. Pergamon Press, Oxford

Brown T (1822) Lectures on the philosophy of the human mind. M. Newman, Andover

Cabanac M (1979) Sensory pleasure. Q Rev Biol 54(1):1–29

Coué É (1923) How to practice suggestion and autosuggestion. American Library Service, New York

Foley TE, Fleshner M (2008) Neuroplasticity of dopamine circuits after exercise: implications for central fatigue. NeuroMol Med 10(2):67–80

Freud S (1929) Introductory lectures on psycho-analysis: a course of twenty eight lectures delivered at the University of Vienna. Allen & Unwin, London

Hoffman R, Hancock P et al (2008) Metrics, metrics, metrics: negative hedonicity. IEEE Intell Syst 23(2):69–73

Houck JR, Duncan A et al (2006) Comparison of frontal plane trunk kinematics and hip and knee moments during anticipated and unanticipated walking and side step cutting tasks. Gait Posture 24(3):314–322

Inglin B, Woollacott M (1988) Age-related changes in anticipatory postural adjustments associated with arm movements. J Gerontol 43(4):M105–M113

Luthe W, Schultz JH (1969) Autogenic therapy. Grune & Stratton, New York

Lyubinskaya S (1970) From stattering to free-flow speech (Rus). Medgiz, Leningrad

Maki BE (1993) Biomechanical approach to quantifying anticipatory postural adjustments in the elderly. Med Biol Eng Comput 31(4):355–362

Nigg BM, Skleryk BN (1988) Clinical Biomechanics 3(2):79–87.

Salter RB (1994) The physiologic basis of continuous passive motion for articular cartilage healing and regeneration. Hand Clin 10(2):211–219

Бернштейн НА (1927) Исследования по биодинамике ходьбы и бега. Труды НТК НКПС вып 63:51–127

Бернштейн НА (1947) О построении движений. Москва, Медгиз

Biomechanics for Life

3

This chapter describes how the floating skeleton concept, which emerged as an academic idea in my biomechanical research, helped me confront some real-world challenges. *Biomechanics for life* grew out of this fortunate application of the concept. The title *biomechanics for life* refers to putting into practice those biomechanical facts and ideas that positively affect our daily activities. I will present here some examples of sanomechanical exercises that can be done without taking time away from other activities. A more structured series is presented in Chap. 4.

3.1
Art of Standing, Sitting, and Walking

It is difficult to stand for a long time. The guards at Buckingham Palace in London, or in the Vatican, or in the Red Square in Moscow change every 15–20 minutes, not because they are bored of being photographed by tourists, but because even young and well-trained men cannot tolerate the associated loads for longer. We need to examine the biomechanical reasons responsible for this sensitivity to static loads in order to develop better strategies for healthy responses to similar, even if less arduous tasks in our daily lives. One of the reasons, as we discussed in Chap. 2, is the high pressure on the joint heads, especially those in the feet. Another reason is that standing creates unfavorable conditions for the sciatic nerves, as we will describe below.

3.1.1
Challenge for Sciatic Nerves

There are two sciatic nerves in our body. They run symmetrically on either side of the base of the spine and pass through the sciatic notches (Fig. 3.1) formed by the ilium bones of the pelvis (Gray and Lewis, 1918). The nerves continue down the thighs, behind our knees, branching out into other nerves in the feet. The sciatic nerves are responsible for the vast amount of sensation generated in the lower body. Pain from muscles, joints, and skin in the area is most likely generated by them.

M.R. Pitkin, *Biomechanics for Life*,
DOI: 10.1007/978-3-642-17177-2_3, © Springer-Verlag Berlin Heidelberg 2011

Fig. 3.1 Sciatic notch in the pelvis. *Red arrow* represents the upper body's weight applied to the Sacrum; *blue arrow* – ground reactions applied to iliac bones from the femur bones (not shown) (Modified from Gray and Lewis (1918) with permission from Bartleby. com, Inc.)

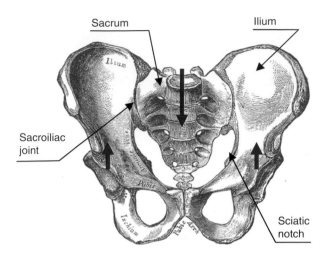

When a person stands on both legs in the "guard" style, with minimal movements of the body segments, the ground reaction is split between the legs equally as shown by the two blue arrows in Fig. 3.1. The arrows are positioned in the areas where the ground reactions are transmitted to the ilium bones through the heads of the femur bones. The weight of the upper body (shown with the red arrow) is transmitted to the pelvis through the sacrum.

Since the ground reactions and the upper body weight are directed in opposite directions but do not act along the same line, they create bending moments relative to each of the two sacroiliac joints (Fig. 3.1). While these joints are not considered as articulated joints, the bending moment, if applied without interruption, creates significant stresses in the area and may cause the sacrum to subside some.

The *floating skeleton* concept explains the mechanism by which the sciatic nerve is irritated and inflamed as follows: if the sacroiliac joints are isolated from the skeleton's hydraulic net for any reason, their cartilages and ligaments[1] will be overstressed. The overstressing may lead to swelling, consequently decreasing the size of the sciatic notch at some point. The process can affect the sciatic nerve and be a source of discomfort and pain.

Having described the biomechanical mechanism for the possible damaging of the sciatic nerves, let us consider two means for preventing such unwanted outcomes. The first one is the activation and restoration of the hydraulic net between joints. A *sanomechanical* approach to this was presented in Chap. 2, and the corresponding exercises will be described below and in Chap. 5.

Here, I would like to focus on the second means for preventing problems associated with the sciatic nerves. This is about our standing and walking styles, and how some of them are be more beneficial to our body than others.

---

[1]*Ligamentum sacroiliacum anterius*, and *ligamentum sacroiliacum posterius* (Gray and Lewis, 1918)

3.1.2
Ancient Standing Style

In ancient sculptures, the standing heroes, athletes, gods, and goddesses usually keep one leg straight and the other slightly bent. The weight of the body is distributed mostly to one leg (Fig. 3.2). We can notice that the pelvis is not kept parallel to the ground, but is tilted toward the flexed leg. The torso has to be bent in the opposite direction (Fig. 3.2b) in order to maintain balance.

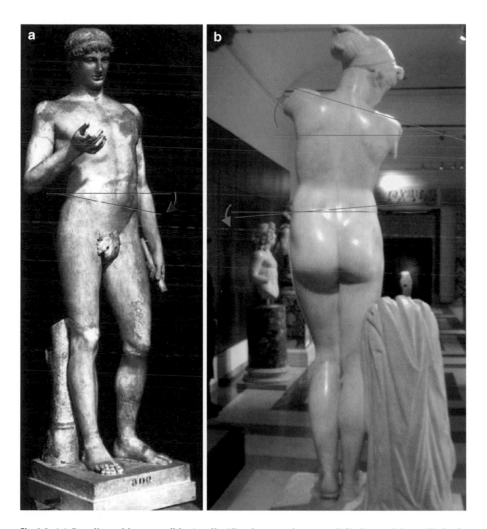

Fig. 3.2 (a) Standing athlete, possibly Apollo (Greek, second century BC), Rome, Museo Torlonia Art. No: ALI176268 EAN-Number: 4050356717875. Adopted with permission; (b) Venere Esquilina (first century AD), Rome, Capitoline Museum. Photograph by the author published with permission

Fig. 3.3 Standing at ease in the gait
laboratory setting. Angle of obliquity is
indicated by *red lines*; the vector of ground
reaction is indicated by the *yellow arrow*
(New England Sinai Hospital Center for
Human Performance, Stoughton, MA)

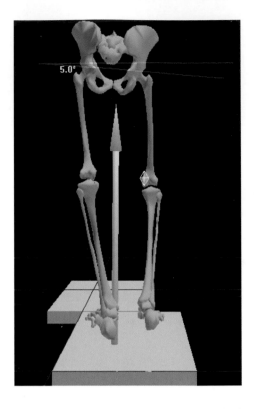

A representation of a standing subject in a "bony" model generated by a computerized
motion analysis permits us to quantify the biomechanical parameters of the tilted pelvis. In
Fig. 3.3, standing *at ease* in a gait laboratory setting is presented. The angle of obliquity
the deviation of the pelvis from the horizontal level in the frontal plane – as well as the
vector of the ground reaction were measured. The angle of obliquity was 5° and is represented by the red arrows; the ground reaction is indicated by the yellow arrow.

When one of the pelvis's sides is not fully supported by the corresponding leg, it can
move down as soon as the muscles holding it parallel to the ground relax. The contacting
surfaces of the femur head and the socket (*acetabulum*) roll relative to one another.

Slow rolling of the acetabulum over the femur head is a good exercise on its own. It can
be qualified as *sanomechanical* if it meets the hedonic criterion of correctness (Chap. 2).
In other words, it has to be driven by a sensation of pleasure and has to be stopped as soon
as the pleasure signal disappears.

People who need to stand for a long time alternate unconsciously between loading one
leg and then the other. They do it to avoid the discomfort or pain from standing on one leg
only. We may say that they use the sanomechanical technique naturally.

During the eleventh of his twelve labors, Heracles[2] fortunately escapes the unbearable
task of holding the sky. Heracles was tasked with bringing golden apples to Eurystheus, but

---

[2]*Library* of Apollodorus, 2.5.11

the golden apples were guarded by the Hesperides, daughters of Atlas, the Titan who held the sky upon his shoulders. Atlas agreed to retrieve the apples if only Hercules would take his place, holding the sky. But when he had received the three apples, Atlas said that he would himself carry the apples to Eurystheus, and that Hercules must hold up the sky forever. By then, Heracles was much exhausted and in severe pain, but managed to trick Atlas to free himself. He asked Atlas to only take the sky again for a few moments while Heracles puts a lion's hide on his shoulders for padding. Atlas agreed and Heracles, triumphant, left him.

The story tells us, besides other things, how difficult it is to stand still on both legs. So we can call Heracles an early adopter of sanomechanics, since his clever wiles stopped the damaging loads on his joints. Such a goal was one that we included in the hedonic criterion of correctness (Chap. 2).

3.2
How Do We Stand?

In the military, keeping personnel in good physical shape is one of the highest priorities. To be ready for any challenges, soldiers undertake extreme training, but not to the extent of damaging the body's integrity. We see this balanced approach in the command *at ease* following the command *at attention*. From an aesthetic point of view, the picture of people in uniform standing *at attention* is quite appealing. However, the military knows how difficult and potentially damaging it would be to hold that rigid position for a long time. The command *at ease* contains very specific instructions on how to load the legs.

The US Army Field Manual teaches that when *at ease*, the body weight has to be applied to one leg: "On the command *at ease*, the soldier may move; however, he must remain standing and silent with his right foot in place."[3]

In the Russian Army, the Field Manual is even more specific. In addition to the US standard, it requires soldiers to alternately relax their legs, and to bend the relaxed leg at the knee.[4]

Nowadays, as in ancient times, there is a collective experience and knowledge about the negative consequences of loading our joints for too long in a static pose, as in symmetrical two-leg standing. Nevertheless, in our daily lives, we often do the opposite.

An example of unnecessary symmetrical two-leg standing is given in Fig. 3.4, where a man is waiting for registration at the airport when a flight delay was announced. The pose provides good stability due to the wide base between his feet. This might be useful in a situation when passersby move quickly and can unintentionally push and destabilize him. However, given the circumstances, when dozens of passengers were standing still for the entire duration of the flight delay, the pose in Fig. 3.4 was not the best one. In this case, a pose of the *at ease* type would be preferable.

---

[3]US Army FM 3-21.5 Drill and Ceremonies
[4]Russian Federation Army FM, 2,28

Fig. 3.4 An example of symmetrical two-leg standing with both knees extended

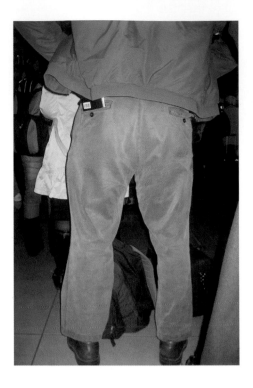

Now I can tell you that I was in the airport when the delay was announced. I knew that standing rigidly, as the passenger on Fig. 3.4, would be too difficult for me, so I stood *at ease*, alternating the load on the legs. I also kept the unloaded relaxed leg bent at the knee, as suggested in the Russian Army Field Manual, or how it was demonstrated by the ancient sculptors in Fig. 3.2. Unfortunately, a second announcement soon came that the flight was again delayed.

I felt tired and my knees and back were sending me signals of discomfort. I walked for a while, but the waiting area was very small and so packed with passengers that there was little space even to walk. So I squatted flat-footedly, with my heels on the floor (Fig. 3.7). It is a stable pose, and allows the body to "sink" while the muscles gradually relax.

For the exercise, I used my sanomechanical technique described in Chap. 2. First, I said to myself as an autosuggestion: "My joints are soaking in synovial liquid and are becoming hydraulically connected." Second, I applied the criterion of correctness of exercises. Namely:

- I sank into a squat through several intermediate positions. The body configuration in each of these positions was "approved" by a sensation of pleasure.
- The duration for holding each of the positions was determined by the disappearance of the pleasure sensation, or by the appearance of a discomfort in any of the joints.

When I began that improvised session, the value and meaning of the flow of the flow of time changed. Focusing on sensations from the depth of the skeleton changed my psychological status. Once only a passenger who was just waiting to board, I became a person consciously and responsively improving his health, even though the situation and environment did not seemingly suit the task. An image formed in my mind of a vessel leaking its vital energy. While exercising, I "felt" that the leaking had stopped.

I can admit that my fellow passengers' initial reaction to my squatting was rather apathetic. As the delay dragged on, more positive attention could be detected. The episode ended when the boarding began, and instead of feeling broken, I felt well and even less tired than when I had arrived at the airport.

3.2.1
Biomechanical Comparison of Free Two-Legged Standing, Standing "at Attention," and Standing "at Ease"

3.2.1.1
Free Standing

A subject (healthy female, 30 years old) was asked to step on the force plates in front of her, stand for a couple of seconds, and step back. In Fig. 3.5, the skeletal lower body model illustrates the initial period when the right leg was swinging and then standing on the right

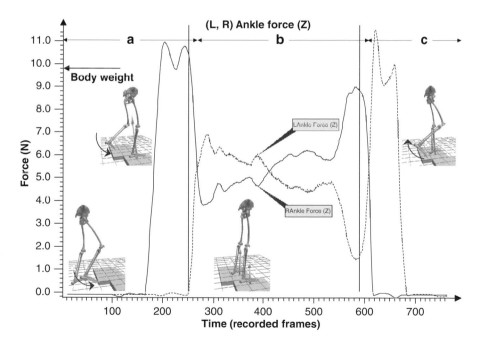

Fig. 3.5 Vertical force on the right (*solid line*) and left (*dotted line*) ankles while: (**a**) stepping on a force plate with the right foot; (**b**) standing on two legs on both force plates; (**c**) lifting the right foot from one force plate, keeping the left foot on the other plate. The *red arrows* indicate the direction in which the corresponding leg is swinging (New England Sinai Hospital Center for Human Performance, Stoughton, MA)

force plate (a); the period of two-legged standing on both force plates (b), the period of one-legged standing when the right foot was removed from the right force plate (c). The graphs in Fig. 3.5 plot the vertical force on the right and left ankles. Similarly to Fig. 1.5, the force is measured in Newtons, normalized to the body weight in kilograms: 9.8 N corresponds to the subject's body weight and is indicated with a black arrow.

Time units are measured by the number of video frames recorded. Since the frequency of recording was 120 Hz, 100 frames correspond to 0.83 s. This gives us an estimate for how long the subject stood just on her right leg (0.80 s), on both force plates with both legs (2.83 s), and the single-leg standing on her left leg (0.58 s).

When the subject was stepping onto the right force plate (a), and until the contralateral leg was in swing, the vertical component of the force on the right ankle replicated the typical pattern of the vertical component of ground reaction seen in the stance period of gait (see Fig. 1.5). Once the two-legged standing on both force plates began (b), we see almost symmetrical waves of force on both ankles, indicating a process of body sway from one leg to another.

The body sway documented in Fig. 3.5b is the natural mechanism of maintaining the dynamic balance of the body while standing, for which the body's entire configuration must change in a coordinated fashion (Thorstensson et al. 1985; Alexandrov et al. 2005; Bottaro 2008). This is why balancing is associated with continuing changes of the loads applied to the contacting bone heads in the joint, and with migration of the zone where the bone heads contact each other.

We may conclude that during free two-legged standing, the migration of the contact zone, together with the change in values of the loads on the joint, provides a means for in-process recovery of the cartilages and other tissues involved in maintaing the body's balance. As long as we agree that the in-process recovery of the loaded tissue depends on how the body maintains balance while standing, we should conclude that any modifications in the style of standing should influence the effectiveness of such recovery.

3.2.1.2
Standing at Attention and at Ease

The two distinct styles that we talked about before were standing *at attention* and *at ease*, for which the loads on the ankle are depicted in Fig. 3.6. When standing at attention (a), both legs were straightened at the knees, as the skeletal model shows. The forces on both ankles plotted in the upper chart are very similar. Unsurprisingly, their values are about half of the body weight, and are kept at the same level without the oscillations seen in free standing (see Fig. 3.5). That means that the body selects a static strategy of maintaining its balance rather than the dynamic strategy observed in free standing. The joints have to be as immobilized as possible, turning the entire body into a single block. We see an example of such immobilization in the graphs of the ankle angle of dorsi/plantarflexion (the lower chart in Fig. 3.6a).

For standing *at ease* (Fig. 3.6b), the forces in ankle joints and the ankle angle of dorsi/plantarflexion are depicted in the upper and lower charts, respectively. The relative position of the body segments is shown with the skeletal model; it replicates those seen in Figs. 3.2 and 3.3.

In this trial, the subject kept most of her weight on her left leg, which is reflected in the high load on the left ankle shown in the red graph.

With this relatively small amount of objective biomechanical data, let us try to explain to ourselves why the *at ease* style is better suited for standing for a long time, compared to the rigid *at attention* style and to the slightly freer two-legged style.

In the *at ease* style we can alternately load and unload the right and left legs, which is not allowed in the *at attention* style. This facilitates in-process recovery, as in the free two-legged style, but when *at ease*, the recovery is more efficient, since the forces on the joints of the unloaded leg are smaller than those in the free two-legged style and significantly smaller than in *at attention* standing.

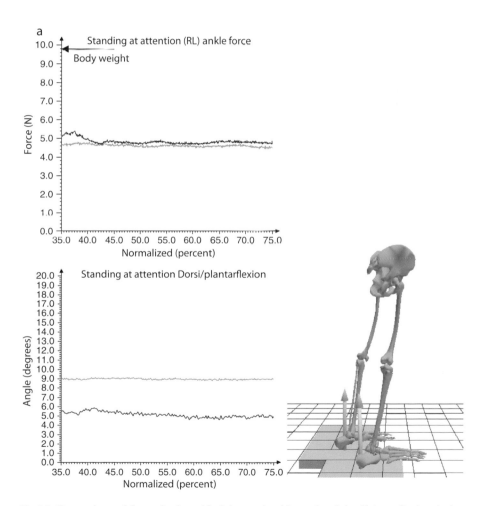

Fig. 3.6 Comparison of forces in the ankle joints and ankle angle of dorsi/plantarflexion during standing *at attention* (**a**) and *at ease* (**b**). Graphs are plotted in green for the right leg and in red for the left leg (New England Sinai Hospital Center for Human Performance, Stoughton, MA)

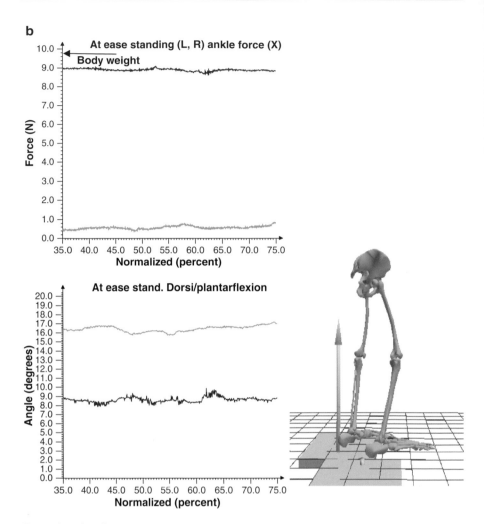

Fig. 3.6 (continued)

3.3
How Do We Sit?

We strain our skeletal system even when we sit. When we are seated, our feet no longer support our body weight. The pelvis, more specifically the lower edges of the *ischium* and *ilium* (see Fig. 3.1), assume that function. The chair exerts pressure against the sensitive soft tissues and skin of the buttocks which are compressed between the seat and the ischium. The seat is so shaped and cushioned as to redistribute the pressures, making them bearable for the compressed soft tissues, which makes sitting comfortable.

While we are seated, the loads that the *sacroiliac joints* and the spine above the *sacrum* experience are comparable to those experienced while standing or walking. The weight of the upper body compresses the lumbar zone of the spine independently of whether we stand or sit. So even though the loads on the ankles, knees, and hips decrease significantly when we sit down, the loads on the lumbar zone remain nearly the same. The rest and recovery process begins for the leg joints, while the spine continues its work against gravity. To reduce the loads on the spine, we put our arms on the desk or on the armrests, lean against our seat back, or recline the seat in search of a more comfortable position.

The problem with sitting comfortably is that we remain motionless for a long time. Consequently, the bone heads in the joints continuously contact each other in the same zones. Since the contacting surfaces of the bone heads are curved, but not congruent, the contact zones have very small areas and the pressures in them are high (see Fig. 1.4). If there is no natural rolling in the joint, and the contact occurs in the same small zone for a long time, the cartilages in the bone heads become overcompressed and may not sufficiently recover from the high pressures, leading to their irreversible destruction.

If we use the same comfortable chair every day at work or another comfortable chair every evening watching television, we will be loading the same combinations of small contacting zones of the joints, raising the risk of their degradation. If the chair is well designed, as in airplanes, we can remain motionless for a long period of time and feel no discomfort. This is a false sensation.

Squatting in the airport was my first public sanomechanical exercise. The experience was a positive one, in terms of how the body felt during and after the performance. I was in a good mood, and not frustrated because of the long delay.

I decided to continue exercising during the flight. The seven hour flight gave ample time to read, have lunch, and do nothing. When I had exhausted this list of activities, I did several exercises shown in Figs. 3.8–3.12.

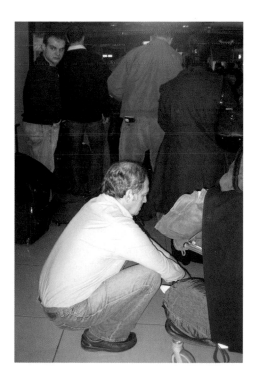

Fig. 3.7 A squat by the author at the airport waiting area during a flight delay

Fig. 3.8 Bending backward on the airplane. Support from the hands for stability. Initial curvature in lumbar zone indicated with blue arc; red arc – painful curvature after articulating in shoulder angle δ and moving belly forward (*blue arrow*)

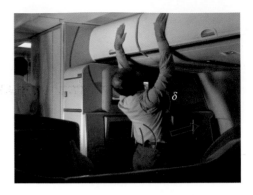

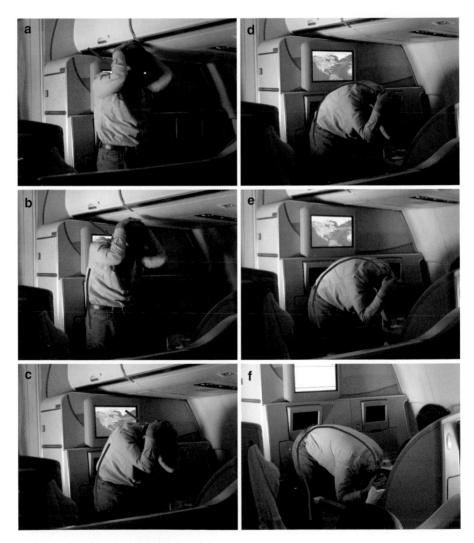

Fig. 3.9 Bending forward: (**a–c**) first half series; (**d–f**) second half series

Fig. 3.10 Twisting the torso as shown with the *white arrows*: (**a**) to the left; (**b**) to the right

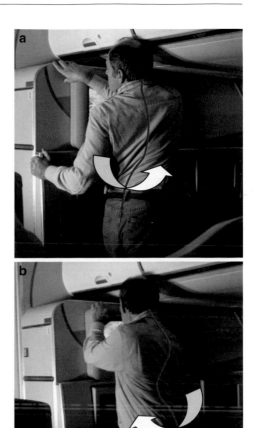

In the first exercise I bent the lumbar zone of the spine backward (Fig. 3.8). It was easy to choose this exercise, considering the many stationary hours spent sitting. In preparation for the pose, I put my hands on the luggage bins for stability. In the initial position shown in Fig. 3.8, my arms were not fully extended at the shoulders, and angle δ of mobility was possible in the sagittal plane. The initial curvature of the lumbar zone is indicated by the blue arc. Since my hands and feet didn't move, it was possible to gradually bend the spine backward, while the belly moved forward as shown with the blue arrow. The red arc indicates the lumbar curvature when the painful sensation occurred for the first time, thereby defining a natural limit for bending further.

I wanted to do this pose and the entire session sanomechanically. Therefore, I focused on the autosuggestion previously used at the flight gate: "My joints are soaked with the synovial liquid and are becoming hydraulically connected." Then, I reminded myself about the criterion of correctness of exercises.

After bending backward the body usually wants to bend forward. For professional gymnasts, and for well-trained people, the ranges of motion in both directions are similar. For me,

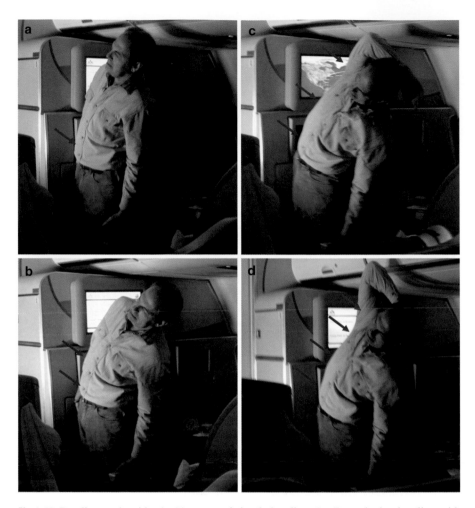

Fig. 3.11 Bending to the side: (**a, b**) stages of simple bending; (**c, d**) continuing bending with lifted arm

the possible amplitude for bending forward was significantly bigger than bending backward. Bending backward required more intermediate positions with coming and disappearing pleasure signals in order to reach the final boundary, beyond which the pain signal made itself known.

The pictures of six consecutive positions (a–f) in forward bending are depicted in Fig. 3.9. You can see that the first three positions (a–c) gave the sensation of encouragement to the bottom of the neck and to the middle of the lumbar zone. Once the transition occurred from position c to position d, the entire neck and back began sending a pleasure signal. The source of that signal was expanding down to the thighs (e) and knees (f). It took about five minutes to make all these transitions. I would have stayed longer in the final position, as the positive sensations hadn't ceased, but I stopped because I felt too much pressure in my head.

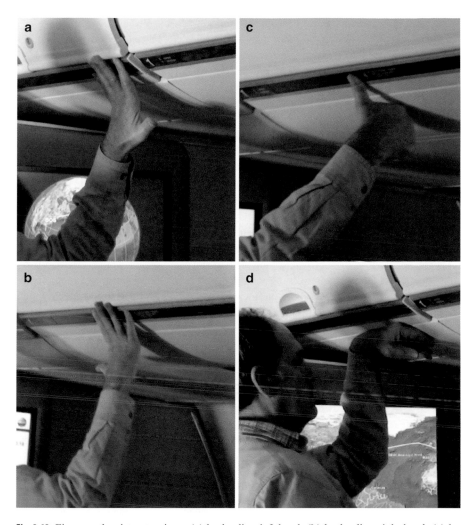

Fig. 3.12 Finger and wrist extensions: (**a**) by loading left hand; (**b**) by loading right hand; (**c**) by loading the thumb; (**d**) by loading the back of the hand

The head cleared when I returned back to position d, which I held for one more minute until the disappearance of the positive sensation in the spine and the back of my legs.

Figure 3.10 depicts a twisting pose, which was performed by rotating the torso to the left (a) and to the right (b). Blue lines along the spine indicate the zones where positive signals (encouraging sensations) were felt. For that pose at that session, I did not need to assume any intermediate positions. Just one motion in either direction was sufficient to stimulate positive signals along the spine.

As I said earlier, this flight was the first one on which I consciously used the sanomechanical technique in exercising. Though I had exercised on almost all previous flights, I could now clearly see a distinction between this sanomechanical technique and the techniques I had used before.

My self-evaluation had already begun at the airport when I filled up the unexciting wait-ing time with one-legged standing and squatting. The fact that I then applied sanomechanical autosuggestion and the criterion of correctness should be considered accidental. I just needed to concentrate on the poses, which looked awkward. Otherwise, I would think only about how I looked to the surrounding passengers. A combination of body configurations selected by the tired body itself, and the conscious methodology which was just a theory before that episode, gave me the inspiration to continue.

After bending the torso in the sagittal plane and twisting it (Figs. 3.8–3.10), it was logi-cal to bend in the frontal plane (Fig. 3.11). By doing this, all three degrees of freedom in the lower back zone were activated.

The series shown in Fig. 3.11. shows bending to the left. The positions a and b cover my range of motion for this zone. But, with the right arm lifted, I could enter two more positions with an expanded amplitude (Fig. 3.11c–d). By adding new blue arrows to the pictures, I am illustrating the expansion of the zone where the sensation of encouragement was detected.

Many flight carriers provide passengers with video instructions on yoga and stretching on the plane. I saw how people would stop reading and chatting, and would start exercising following the video instructions. From that point of view, the plane is a psychologically more suitable and friendly place for your own routine, even if you perform it alone – which is why on that flight, historic for me, I felt comfortable enough to make two more series: for hands and for feet.

Afflicted by arthritis in my hands, I had felt stiffness build up in my fingers and wrist, which I sought to alleviate. The hand series is briefly illustrated in Fig. 3.12, where pic-tures a through c show extension of the fingers, and d illustrates wrist flexion.

The last exercise was a combination of knee and foot flexion (Fig. 3.13). The pose in the picture is self-explanatory with obvious advantages for the legs after extended sitting. It is interesting that the motion of the foot in the ankle joint, which is shown in the picture, is called

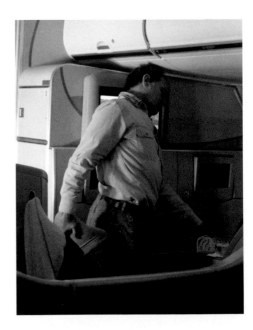

Fig. 3.13 Simultaneous flexion in the knee and the foot

"flexion." The nuance is that by definition, flexion is an articulation in a joint which shortens the limb. Here, the foot motion elongates the leg and should be called "extension." The confusion arises because in humans, the default orientation of the foot relative to the shin constitutes 90°, versus 0° for the hand's orientation. However, flexion in the wrist goes in the direction of the inwardly curved palm; the motion we are discussing in the foot goes in the direction of the downward pointing sole, which is the anatomical equivalent of the palm. A convention was established to call this motion "flexion" or "plantarflexion," because of the anatomical closeness between the foot and the hand.

Here I shared with you a selection of the poses that I wanted to maintain, because of the powerful response my body sent in the form of a pleasant sensation. I interpret that sensation as my body's encouraging me to maintain those positions. I can explain the biomechanical process that the body wants me to initiate with the poses. And the explanation is that by holding the poses with the signal of pleasure control, we help the body to restore and activate the hydraulic net of the skeletal joints.

The selection of poses for conducting a series of sanomechanical exercises has to be very much individual, depending on your particular needs in different body parts.

3.4
How Do We Walk?

The "heel-on" event at each step marks the moment when the foot finishes its travel through the air (swing phase) and touches the ground. The initial contact of the foot with the ground generates so-called *transient*[5] *forces* which are transmitted through the skeleton up to the head. On the graphs of the ground reaction and forces in the joints, the transient has the shape of a peak followed by a brief decline. An example of such peaks can be seen at 3% of the stride in Fig. 1.5, where the forces on the ankle, knee, and hip joints are plotted along with the ground reaction force. Larger transient forces are recorded during unusual or unexpected conditions on the ground, for instance, due to unknown surface height (van der Linden et al. 2009).

By observing the transient we may better appreciate the discovery of the ancient thinkers that gait is a well organized cyclic sequence of falls. We will delve deeper into their and their followers' ideas in Chap. 5, where we will discuss what "well" organized means in relation to the body falls. Here I would like to bring your attention to the word "organized" as a generic term applicable to the structure of any process. As such, the term presumes that someone or something is responsible for the job of organizing the process in all respects: formulating a task, prioritizing and synchronizing, and controlling its execution. If "something" is Mother Nature, we usually give the highest merit to the job. But when the responsibility is delegated to human consciousness, we reasonably accept that the work of organizing can be imperfect, not good, or even quite poor.

The latter is the case for gait as an organized process of falls. Since Mother Nature gives us a tangible share in motion control, the gait indeed may be organized with different levels of quality. While the quality of gait can also be defined differently, we will be talking about quality from the point of view of maintaining and prolonging the health of the skeleton.

---

[5]*Transient* = passing especially quickly into and out of existence

Returning to transient forces, we should recognize that they may be more or less harmful, with a variety of pathological outcomes like headaches, degenerative joint disease, and stress fractures (Folman et al. 1986; Whittle 1999). If the excessive cyclic transient forces are dangerous, can we do anything to lower the risk associated with daily walking?

3.4.1
Indian Gait and Ballet Gait

In 2010, a study was conducted at the Center for Human Performance of the New England Sinai Hospital to compare biomechanical characteristics associated with the regular gait style and two special styles. I selected these styles after reading a paper by Dr. Harris published in 1914 in the *Military Surgeon* journal (Harris 1914), and a more recent book by Dr. Ashton (Ashton 1986). Dr. Harris, in his work, gave a description of the gait practiced by Native American Indians, indicating its positive aspects for the body. The term *Indian gait* relates to the walking style once practiced not only by American Indians, but also by barefoot natives in the tropics and Eskimos in the polar regions. The key determinants of Indian gait are the straight pointing of the toes and the toe–heel sequence in the foot contact with the ground. The latter was suggested as a means to walk with less noise, which was essential for hunting, compared to the *regular* gait with the heel–toe sequence (Macfarlan 1971). Since noise level can be taken as a measure of the transient, it seemed interesting to discover whether a difference between Indian and regular gait styles could be objectively documented.

The second gait style for comparison with regular gait was *ballet gait*, which mimics the stage walking style of ballet dancer. The toes are oriented notably outward, where the orientation of the foot is relative to the line of body progression (angle of foot progression). A positive number corresponds to an internally rotated foot (Fig. 3.14).

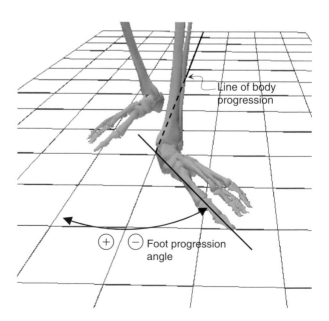

Fig. 3.14 Convention regarding the angle of foot progression: a positive number corresponds to an internally rotated foot

Fig. 3.15 Conventions regarding the angles in knee and ankle: (**a**) positive number corresponds to knee flexion, negative number corresponds to knee extension; (**b**) positive number corresponds to ankle dorsiflexion, negative number corresponds to ankle plantarflexion

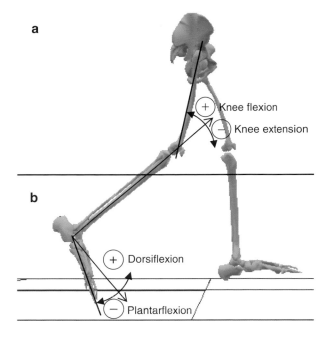

Dr. Aston observed that there was a link between the angle of progression and the flexion/extension function of the knee during weight bearing (Ashton 1986). He explained that with an excessive angle of foot progression, the knee is less able to flex during weight bearing. The reason is that with the excessive outward positioning of the foot, the entire leg rotates outward at the hip joint. The knee joint, as shown in Fig. 3.15, has a single axis of articulation for flexion/extension, and that axis lies in the frontal plane of the body (perpendicularly to the line of progression). The excessive outward rotation of the leg turns the axis of the knee joint toward the line of progression. The closer the axis is to the line of progression, the more difficult it is to flex or extend the knee during the stance period. Since the stance knee flexion/extension with an amplitude of approximately 15° is one of the key characteristics of regular gait – it provides shock absorption during load bearing of body weight (Perry 1992) – the decrease of the knee angulation could be a negative attribute of ballet gait.

Thus, the comparative biomechanical study was designed to compare regular, Indian, and ballet gait styles. Prior to the study, the Institutional Review Board of the New England Sinai Hospital approved the protocol and the informed consent form.

3.4.2
Comparative Gait Study

Seven sound volunteers aged 22–25 agreed to participate in the study after each had read and signed the consent form. They were asked to walk along a 10-m walkway with two embedded force plates (Kistler). The subjects walked with the regular heel–toe sequence, repeating the trials four times, and with the Indian style toe–heel sequence, also repeating the trial four times.

We used the angle of ankle dorsi/plantarflexion as the single kinematic parameter of distinction between the regular and Indian styles, though with a clear understanding that the original Indian gait can be organized in a more complicated fashion than described by Dr. Harris. Walking with the toe–heel sequence, however, is not an absolutely new task, since we always practice it when walking down stairs. After few attempts, all subjects were able to walk with the Indian style quite easily.

The subjects were then asked to walk with ballet gait, positioning their feet on the ground more outwardly than in regular gait. The subjects were not aware of the expectations regarding possible connections between the style-defining parameters and other biomechanical characteristics.

3.4.2.1
Indian Gait Outcomes

Fig. 3.16 depicts a comparison of the vertical ground reaction (GR) and forces on the joints during regular (graphs in red color, previously shown in Fig. 1.5) and Indian (graphs in blue color) gait. The transients registered in regular gait are indicated by the

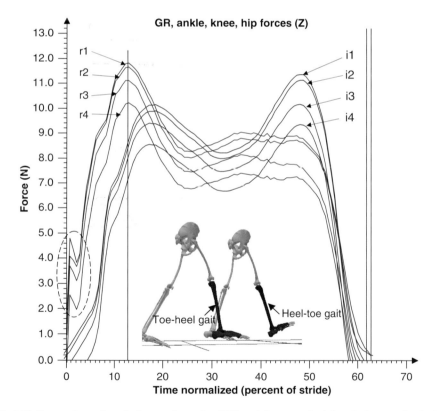

Fig. 3.16 Comparison of vertical ground reaction (*GR*) and forces on the joints during regular (*red*) and Indian gait (*blue*). Regular gait parameters: r1 - ground reaction; r2 – ankle; r3 – knee; r4 – hip. Indian gait: i1 - ground reaction; i2 – ankle; i3 – knee; i4 – hip (New England Sinai Hospital Center for Human Performance, Stoughton, MA)

dashed oval. In Indian gait the transients did not appear. The first maxima in all forces were also smaller in Indian gait compared to the regular style.

The absence of the transient peaks during the foot foot-on event, illustrated in Fig. 3.16, is an objective supporting argument in favor of Dr. Harris's suggestion that it is the toe–heel sequence which decreases the impact from the initial load bearing, and therefore makes the Indian style of gait less noisy and more healthy (Harris 1914).

3.4.2.2
Ballet Gait Outcomes

Analysis of data obtained from ballet gait showed a notable decrease in the knee flexion during stance phase (Fig. 3.17). Instead of the flexion observed in regular gait, the knee hyper-extends.

We can also see that the amplitude of the knee angle is about five times less than in regular gait. That tells us that the relative rolling of the femur and tibial bone heads, which is needed for shock absorption, is almost absent in ballet gait.

3.4.3
How Do We Walk? Conclusions

It would be too simplistic to recommend that people walk with the toe–heel sequence. Although we demonstrated that it may decrease the negative consequences of impact during load bearing, it is impractical and risky to relearn how to walk. Nevertheless, we can say that it is also not correct to neglect the long-term consequences of the transients to joint health.

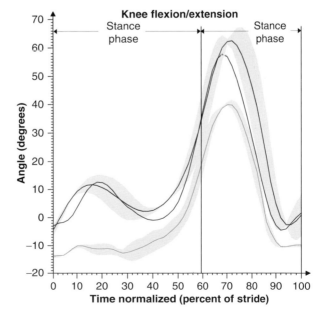

Fig. 3.17 Knee dorsi/plantarflexion angle (defined in Fig. 3.15) during stance phase of regular (*red*), Indian (*blue*) and ballet (*green*) styles of gait. Shadowed areas represent one standard deviation from the average values (New England Sinai Hospital Center for Human Performance, Stoughton, MA)

Refraining from excessive outward positioning of the foot cannot be bluntly recommended either. This characteristic is only one component of the real style adopted by professional ballet dancers during many years of multifaceted training. When you watch them moving across the stage, you can see that in addition to the high value of the foot progression angle they also use the toe–heel sequence, which we attributed here to the Indian gait. More studies are needed to learn if that positive component of reducing the transients by using the toe–heel sequence would compensate for the negative component of hyperextension in the knees due to excessive outward positioning of the foot.

I believe that understanding the issue of transients and knee shock absorption function can prevent us from irresponsibly dropping our body weight with every step.

My angle of foot progression is not excessive, and I use the heel–toe sequence, but when I instruct myself "I am walking noiselessly," the level of noise somehow diminishes. Mother Nature is helpful if we ask specifically and if the request is rational.

Unfortunately, it is not easy to change the daily routine. However, when we hear from a friend at a school reunion "Look at you. You haven't changed!" – it is our daily routine which will determine whether the friend's words are true, or just motivated by traditional politeness.

3.5
We Do Not Need a Special Time to Do Sanomechanical Exercises

Routine recovery means performing pleasure-driven exercises during short time intervals in the daily interactions with environment. Doing it during your working hours without compromising your performance is an excellent complimenting component to your natural recovery when you sleep. It increases your productivity and self-confidence, and allows you to think and care more about people you love.

The best time for sanomechanical exercises is when you cannot avoid waiting for something. You are familiar with such situations very well, since they happen every day. Let me give you some examples of what can be done, and you will be able to expand the list indefinitely based on your own schedule.

3.5.1
Computers

Working with computers gives us several "free" minutes when the computer is being turned on, or when large files or programs are loaded. That is the best time for doing one or two poses for your neck.

- Close your eyes and say to yourself: "My neck is hydraulically connected to the entire skeleton. It is flexible, strong, and ever young."
- Bend the neck in either plane until the first positive signal appears. Hold it until that signal disappears.
- Return the head to the neutral position.

You are done for now. Resume your work, and be prepared to use the next good moment for the next pose(s).

3.5.2
Car

The correct use of a car is a safe transition from point A to point B. A driver needs to be biomechanically prepared to quickly respond to any unexpected situation. The time period between the signal and the response has to be at its absolute minimum. The mechanism controlling that period is called *anticipation*.

When the nervous system actively anticipates possible challenges, it reacts faster and more efficiently. It generates the best programs for controlling coordinated movements of the body, which is a system with multiple degrees of freedom. This makes the autosuggestion an instrument in the biomechanical "toolbox." We discussed it in Chap. 2, when we spoke about *sanomechanical autosuggestion*. Thus,

- a sanomechanical suggestion before you turn on the ignition is: "I am going to ...*name of a destination*, and I am in control of the situation on the road and around."

When you stop at a gas station and wait for your tank to fill, you may do a bending or twisting exercise of your choice (Fig. 3.18).

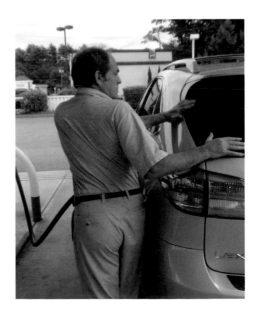

Fig. 3.18 Twisting the torso outside the car at a gas station

3.5.3
Shopping

Almost every shopping trip is associated with several minutes of waiting. Let us make them the best minutes of a day. It is possible if you make couple of sanomechanical exercises with positive sensations (Fig. 3.19).

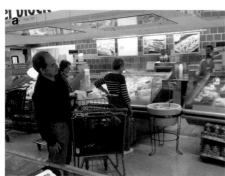
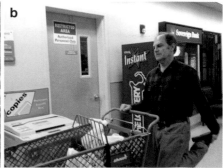

Fig. 3.19 Exercising while shopping: (**a**) bending to the side; (**b**) knee and foot flexing

3.5.4
Museum

Going to an exhibit can make you very tired, but it should not. A biomechanical reason behind the extra tiredness in a museum is the slow walking with interruption for standing still in front of paintings and other art objects. As we will see in Chap. 5, slow gait requires more energy than gait with self-selected speed. The latter is the most energy-efficient pace because of the ballistic mechanisms of gait are utilized. Also, standing and walking slowly increase the contact time between the bone heads in the joints. That stresses joint cartilages, especially if the synovial capsules do not have a sufficient amount of synovial liquid and if the hydraulic connectivity between the joints is broken.

I suggest using some sanomechanical poses while looking at objects of interest, as shown in Fig. 3.20.

I have now included these poses in my routine of attending all professional meetings, exhibitions, and shows. It helps me leave the events without being physically exhausted, as I used to before discovering sanomechanics. At some gatherings, with all the people around me, I don't feel psychologically comfortable doing the exercises when my body requires. In these cases, I try to find a less crowded area and do some sanomechanics anyway. One should remember his/her hierarchy of priorities, and use more *ego* and *super ego* for protecting the *id* as we discussed in Chap. 2.

In conclusion, I will suggest a quiz for you. Please look at the pictures of two of the visitors of the museum, who are looking at the same painting, but in different poses (Fig. 3.21). Who do you think will be more tired afterward?

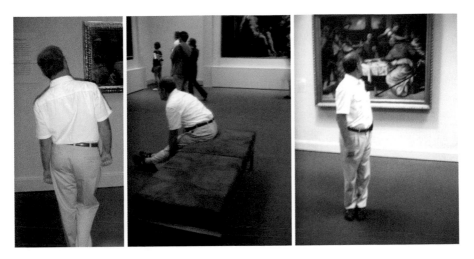

Fig. 3.20 Useful poses for museum

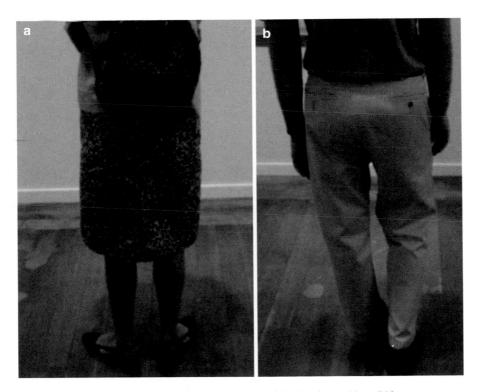

Fig. 3.21 Who will be more tired after the museum: the visitor in picture (**a**) or (**b**)?

3.6
Conclusion

We have considered basic locomotor functions: standing, walking and sitting, and their contribution to our daily activities. We pointed out the risk posed by any of these activities if they are performed with a body configuration that remains unchanged for a long time. The main risk factor is the high local pressure applied to the contacting zones of the joint's heads, which deforms cartilage. An additional risk factor is the misleading sensory information about the factual pressures, preventing us from detecting the overpressure sooner.

Let us go back to Fig. 1.4 (Li et al. 2008) showing the compressive cartilage contact deformation distributions at different time intervals after loading. The picture demonstrates that after 20 s of standing still, the indent in the cartilage is already as big as after 300 s. However, after standing still for 20 s, a healthy person does not feel the warning sensations alerting him that the layer of cartilage is fully compressed. The warning sensation might appear in several minutes, leaving the joint heads excessively overloaded.

Now we know about this risk and will try avoiding still postures by using more rolling motions in the joints and changing our body configurations consciously. Another protective measure would be to increase preparedness of the skeleton to the unavoidable overloading by including sanomechanics exercises in our daily routine.

References

Alexandrov AV, Frolov AA et al (2005) Feedback equilibrium control during human standing. Biol Cybern 93(5):309–322

Ashton R (1986) Fundamental system: bad feet – bad spine. Society of Metaphysicians Limited

Bottaro A, Yasutake Y et al (2008) Bounded stability of the quiet standing posture: an intermittent control model. Hum Mov Sci 27(3):473–495

Folman Y, Wosk J et al (1986) Cyclic impacts on heel strike: a possible biomechanical factor in the etiology of degenerative disease of the human locomotor system. Arch Orthop Trauma Surg 104(6):363–365

Gray H, Lewis WH (1918) Anatomy of the human body. Lea & Febiger, Philadelphia, Bartleby. com, 2000. www.bartleby.com/1–7/

Harris J (1914) Falt feet – the etiological relations of posture and gait tereto. Mil. Surg. 34(1):1–11

Li G, Wan L, Kozanek M (2008) Determination of real-time in-vivo cartilage contact deformation in the ankle joint. J Biomech 41(1):128–136

Macfarlan AA (1971) Modern hunting with Indian secrets; basic, old-new skills for observing and matching wits with nature. Stackpole Books, Harrisburg

Perry J (1992) Gait analysis: normal and pathological function. Slack, Inc., Thorofare

Thorstensson A, Oddsson L et al (1985) Motor control of voluntary trunk movements in standing. Acta Physiol Scand 125(2):309–321

van der Linden MH, Hendricks HT et al (2009) Hitting a support surface at unexpected height during walking induces loading transients. Gait Posture 29(2):255–260

Whittle MW (1999) Generation and attenuation of transient impulsive forces beneath the foot: a review. Gait Posture 10(3):264–275

Sanomechanics™ Exercises

4

4.1
Introduction Regarding Safety

Sanomechanical exercises are those poses which activate hydraulic connectivity between skeleton joints. Each pose focuses on a selected degree or degrees of freedom. The purpose of each pose is to enact a certain body configuration appreciated by the body within these degrees of freedom. That appreciation is conveyed by our nervous system as a sensation of pleasure, which is sent to the mind as a signal of encouragement. Unwanted deviations from the correct poses evoke a signal of discouragement (pain), instructing us to adjust the pose.

Trust yourself. Be confident that when the body sends a pleasant signal evoked by a certain pose, it wants to encourage you to maintain that pose and prolong the signal with new positions. Use the waves of the encouragement signals (Fig. 2.5) to guide you from position to position. Based on the pictures of the suggested exercises in this chapter, develop your own routine, reflecting your individual particularities and needs.

You now understand the nature of encouraging and discouraging signals, and know how to use them, how to control the correctness of the poses and their duration, and how to maintain safety and maximize positive outcomes. Remember, an exercise is performed to increase the body's preparedness for those loads and disturbances of balance that could otherwise be damaging. So the loads associated with exercises should not exceed those for which the body is not yet prepared. We should always listen carefully and analyze the signals that our sensors generate.

4.2
Make Your Morning

Every morning, the transition from the horizontal to the vertical position constitutes a serious task for all organs and systems of the waking body. In the vertical position, the body has to deal with the maximal effect of gravity, in contrast to gravity's minimal effect in the horizontal position. Even for a person in good health, the first step after bed may cause a sprain of the ankle, Achilles tendon, or knee ligaments. A high percentage of elderly

M.R. Pitkin, *Biomechanics for Life*,
DOI: 10.1007/978-3-642-17177-2_4, © Springer-Verlag Berlin Heidelberg 2011

people's falls happen in the morning in the first minutes after bed. Proper preparation for the transition between sleep and wakefulness can eliminate many potential problems, including immediate injuries.

If you feel stiffness or pain in the joints of your legs or in your torso when you wake up, it is a direct indication that the transition to a vertical position can be risky. Preparatory exercises while in bed are the correct response to this situation. They prepare the body for the high loads associated with vertical posture in the field of gravity.

Autosuggestion, which comprises the intellectual part of the sanomechanical technique, activates the nervous control system, "telling" it what to expect. In return, the nervous system becomes "aware" of the anticipated task, for example of maintaining balance, and responds optimally to unexpected tasks like avoiding obstacles in the course of locomotion and other physical activities. Autosuggestions in the morning before waking up entirely are most effective, since a relaxed body provides the highest suggestibility for the mind.

4.3
Why Are My Joints Stiffer After I Sleep?

Since you are familiar by now with the floating skeleton concept, you can see that your morning stiffness and soreness can be explained by insufficient hydraulic connectivity between the joints. The mechanism of hydraulic connectivity is capillarity. The instruments of this mechanism are osmosis and the deformation of the synovial capsules. When we sleep at night, we are drying out, and osmosis may not deliver a sufficient amount of fluid to the space between the bones and the periosteum. The capsules' "pump" may also not work well if we do not change body position for a long time. Joint inflammation, for example due to arthritis, causes morning stiffness and pain because the body treats inflammation with edema, fluid outflow that is retained in the synovial capsule. The pressure increases in the affected capsule and blocks the hydraulic connectivity with the neighboring joints' capsules.

Usually, the hands and feet are the first body parts that experience morning stiffness. The periosteum's "gloves" and "socks" have to deliver synovial fluid to many joints of small bones whose shape is complex, and which may lie at the end of delivery routes more fragile than those to long bones.

4.4
The Difference Between Exercising on a Yielding and a Firm Surface

I am going to show you several sanomechanical exercises which I developed for myself to avoid beginning my day with arthritis pain medications. I developed these exercises after I failed to complete regular yoga exercises in a class because of pain.

From the point of view of mechanics, the difference between performing yoga poses on a firm floor and in bed is in the degree to which skeletal arcs straighten. In Fig. 4.1, a low back arc of the spine is simulated with four pivotally connected blocks. The blocks move down under gravity and spread horizontally (Fig. 4.2). With support under the initial arc that simulates a soft yielding surface like a mattress (Fig. 4.2a), the spine flattens less than on the firm surface (Fig. 4.2b).

The simulation explains why a firm surface is necessary to better straighten the spine's curves, and to more effectively extend stiff joints. However, in order to reach your exercise mat on the floor, you have to leave bed, which, if done unprepared, can be risky. You should therefore first prepare your body by doing sanomechanical exercises while in bed. For those readers who avoid yoga because of discomfort and pain during exercising on a firm surface, the sanomechanical series in bed will be an excellent gateway.

Exercising in bed does not substitute exercising on firm surfaces and while standing. It is not a substitute for any workout you are interested in doing this or any other day. What it does is complete the revitalization of the hydraulic net in your skeleton – a vitalization which was supposed to be completed during the night's sleep, but for some reason was not finalized by the time you woke up this morning.

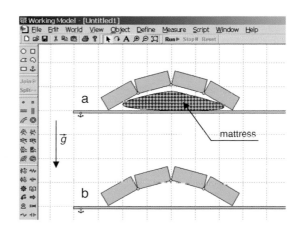

Fig. 4.1 Initial position of a flexible arc on a soft (**a**) and firm (**b**) support. Working Model simulation

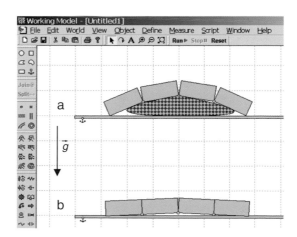

Fig. 4.2 Flattening of the flexible arc (see Fig. 4.1) under gravity on the soft (**a**) and firm (**b**) surfaces. Working Model simulation

4.5
Sanomechanical In-Bed Series

4.5.1
Hand and Foot Poses

4.5.1.1
Extending Fingers and Wrists

We start with the hands and feet for two reasons. First, because these body parts are designed with about 30 degrees of freedom, each of which can be a source of discomfort and pain if kept unused. Second, we begin the sanomechanical series immediately after waking up, and even before we waking up entirely. This is a precious time we want to extend, and more active movements would be too aggressive for the body and the mind.

You have the choice of beginning with a pose devoted to extension or flexion in the fingers and the wrists. I suggest doing extensions first, because these movements are usually discriminated against during our daily routine. Indeed, our hands' most frequent movements are different grasps. That leaves some areas of the joints' heads unused.

So, here is the extension series for the fingers and wrists (Fig. 4.3). The initial pose is shown in Fig. 4.3a, with fingers spread against the headboard. Once you find a comfortable position of the wrist that gives you a positive sensation, you can keep it for several minutes, still without fully waking up.

Go to position "b" when position "a" stops generating encouraging signals. From there, you can reach the final position "d" with one or more intermediate positions like position "c." You might sense a positive signal in all your fingers or just in one. Above all, be careful to avoid the negative signal of discouragement or pain. It is also assumed that lying on your belly is comfortable enough. Otherwise, you should change to a better body position.

You can see from the photographs in Fig. 4.3b–d that the wrist's extension angle gradually increases. Moving from "a" to "d" usually takes me about 5 min, but if I feel more stiffness in the fingers, I do these extensions for longer. Here and in all other exercises, one should follow the principle of *quantum satis*.[1]

If you indeed find the pleasant zone(s) for the fingers and the wrists, it is quite possible that you will fall asleep again with your hands in one of the poses "a"–"d." It is also possible that a pleasant sensation will be generated in your shoulders and/or elbow joints. In any case, you will figure out that it is time to go to the flexion poses for the fingers and the wrists which you just extended so nicely.

---

[1]*Quantum satis* is a Latin term meaning "the amount which is needed." Pharmacists use it to indicate how much solvent should be added when blending a mixture until it reaches the desired consistency

Fig. 4.3 Finger and wrist extensions. (**a**) Positioning of the palms on the headboard; (**b**) sliding alongside the torso to the first encouraging position; (**c**) next encouraging position; (**d**) final encouraging position

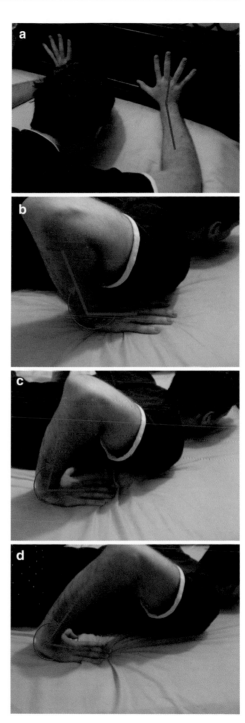

4.5.1.2
Flexing Fingers and Wrists

The initial pose for the flexion series in the wrist is shown in Fig. 4.4a, with an almost fully extended wrist angle. As with the extension series, once you find an initial position of the wrist that gives you a positive sensation, you may maintain it for several minutes.

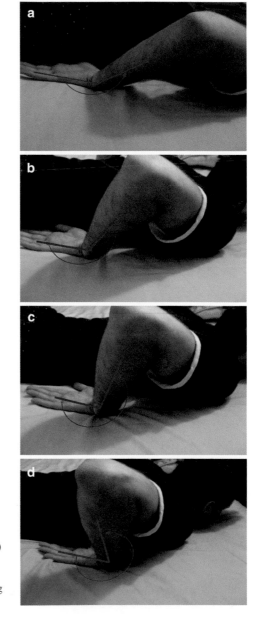

Fig. 4.4 Wrist bending exercises.
(**a**) Positioning of the palms (dorsal aspect) on the bed; (**b**) sliding alongside the torso to the first encouraging position; (**c**) next encouraging position; (**d**) final encouraging position

Change to position "b" when position "a" stops generating encouraging signals. You should ultimately reach the final position "d," passing through one or more intermediate positions like position "c." As in all other positions, you need to avoid the negative signal of discouragement or pain.

The initial pose for the flexion series in the fingers is shown in Fig. 4.5a.

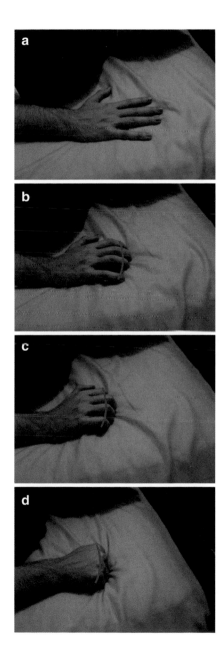

Fig. 4.5 Finger flexion exercises.
(**a**) Positioning of the palms on the bed; (**b**) gradually flexing the fingers to the first encouraging position; (**c**) next encouraging position; (**d**) final encouraging position

4.5.2
Toe and Foot Poses

Toe and foot poses are shown in Fig. 4.6. When a position with an encouraging sensation for toe flexion (Fig. 4.6a) or extension is found, we hold it with our muscles relaxed. That allows gravity to slowly work against resistance from ligaments and synovial membranes. Blue arcs show areas where the encouraging sensation might be more noticeable.

Inversion and eversion are very important degrees of freedom for the feet. Insufficient mobility (laxity) in the ankle-subtalar-joint complex can be the reason for ligament sprains and even ruptures (Nigg, et al. 1990). When the foot lands on rough terrain, rather than on a flat horizontal surface, the vector of ground reaction may develop a moment relative to the contact point of the tibia and talar bones. The more everted or inverted the orientation of the foot relative to the shin, the larger the moment will be from the ground reaction, and the more challenging the load applied to the ligaments will be.

Doing morning exercises in the ankle-subtalar complex is a good preventive measure for the first steps out of bed, and a good preparation for the day's activities.

4.5.3
Knee and Hip Closed Poses

From a supine position, we begin bending one leg at the knee (Fig. 4.7a). The other leg follows, and we fully wrap the legs with our arms (Fig. 4.7b–d). Note that in the position shown in Fig. 4.7d, both the knee and the hip joints generate encouraging sensations.

After the positive sensations in the knees and hips disappear, we slowly extend the knees (Fig. 4.7e, f) until sensation of encouragement reaches the area behind the knees (Fig. 4.7g).

When the sensation in the knees disappears, we slowly swing both legs to the right of the torso (Fig. 4.7h).

You can appreciate the importance of this position by the high level of positive sensation in the hips. Strong encouragement for practicing this pose has anatomical justification. The relative orientation of the legs and the pelvis in this position is extremely rare in our daily life. Therefore, the zones of the head of the femur bone and the socket (*acetabulum*), which form the hip joint, are underused. That passivity is responsible for the insufficient delivery of synovial liquid to other pelvic joints. The first beneficiaries of the exercise in Fig. 4.7h will be the three joints forming the socket of the hip joint where three bones (*ilium, ischium, pubis*) come together (Fig. 3.1).

4.5.4
Spine and Pelvis Poses

Twenty four vertebrae are assembled in the spine, with different predetermined ranges of motion. The upper seven (cervical) vertebrae and lower five (lumbar) vertebrae are quite

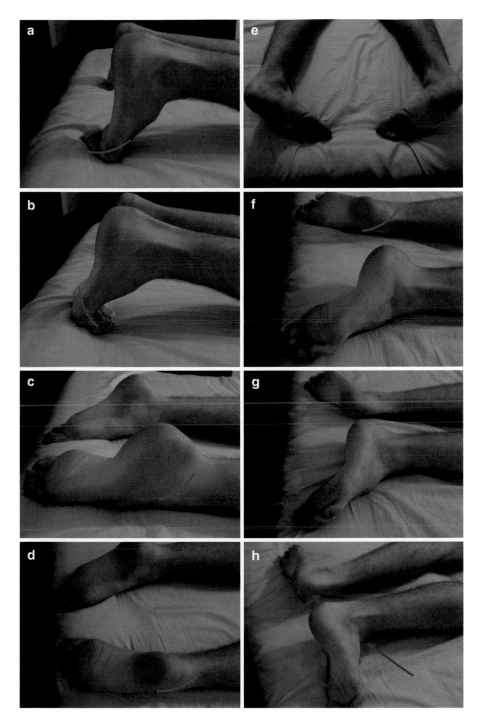

Fig. 4.6 Toe and foot exercises. (**a**) Gradually flexing the toes to the first encouraging position; (**b**) positioning the toes upon the bed for extension under gravity; (**c–e**) gradually inverting the feet; (**f–h**) gradually everting the feet

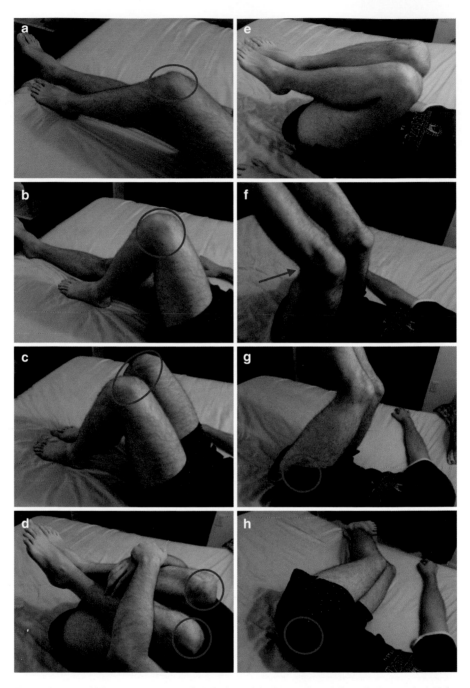

Fig. 4.7 Knee and hip poses: (**a**–**d**) gradual flexion of the knees; (**e** and **f**) gradual extension of the knees; (**g** and **h**) twisting parallel legs at the hip joints

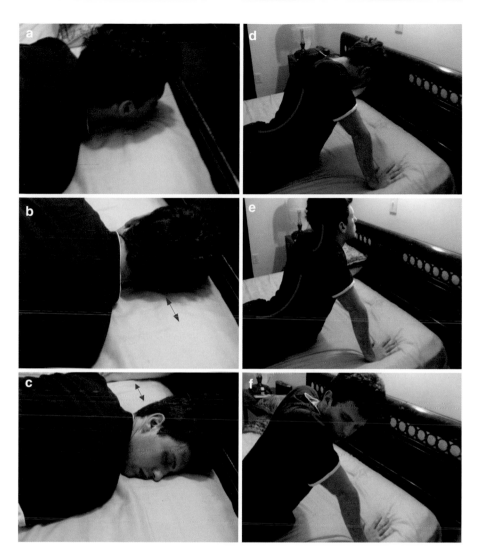

Fig. 4.8 Poses for the neck and for extension of the back

movable, but the middle twelve (thoracic vertebrae, connected to the ribs) are mostly immobile. Vertebrae are connected to each other by intervertebral disks, so the joints of the spine are not synovial, but of the cartilaginous type. Pelvic joints are also not synovial, being of the fibrous type, and under normal circumstances, pelvic bones do not move.

Even though the joints of the spine and pelvis are not synovial, I believe that they are also included in the hydraulic net, like the synovial joints in the arms and legs. In performing the sanomechanical exercises for the spine and pelvis, I do not see any differences in the dynamic of sensation described in Chap. 2. Moreover, application of the criterion of correctness and autosuggestion focused on the spine and pelvis have brought to me the most notable positive effects.

As we see everywhere in the body, the organs, systems, and tissues that are not put to use in their full capacity steadily degrade and atrophy. For the spine and pelvis, the negative consequences of immobility are very serious, due to the biomechanical role of both cervical and lumbar parts. Mobility in the lumbar part is a key component of normal gait synergy (Pitkin 2009). If mobility in this zone is restricted due to lower back pain, normal ballistic synergy is substituted by compensatory movements of the body segments, with a consequently greater energy expenditure and smaller aesthetics of locomotion (Perry 1992).

We begin by focusing on the cervical part of the spine by supporting the chin (Fig. 4.8a). The blue arrow shows the possible initial positions of the chin. It reminds us that the very first position for the pose should be selected with the criterion of correctness in mind. A search for the correct placement of the chin has to be very slow, and gentle with respect to the spine. Once a pleasant sensation appears, we hold the initial pose for a while, and then carefully follow the dynamic of sensation.

As soon as the pleasant sensation disappears, we may want to try the next position with the chin's support, or may want to pass to the turned head position (Fig. 4.8b). The blue arrow, as in position a, shows that it may be necessary to try several initial positions before the encouragement signal from the upper region of the spine can be detected.

After completing exercise b, we go to exercise c, where the head is turned to the other side.

It may seem odd that positions a–c are the same that the body had maintained for several hours while you slept. They are not the same, and will bring you benefit, since these exercises are performed without the elevation of a pillow. You will immediately feel a different sensation in the neck as soon as the pillow is removed. That will be true even if you sleep on a very thin pillow.

Now we are ready for extension poses for the spine. Bend upward, as shown in Fig. 4.8d–f. In position d, we may combine the extension of the spine in the lumbar zone with flexion in the cervical zone. The latter occurs under gravity, as the neck muscles are gradually relaxed. That relaxation can be done very carefully and gradually indeed.

After completing pose d, we may go to e and f, which differ from pose d in the positioning of the head. To support the head in these poses, the neck muscles cannot be fully relaxed, so we carefully try to maintain a balance between their and gravity's action.

Positions d–f are the first exercises which require some muscular effort, similar to those needed for the turn in bed. If you feel that these loads exceed your morning conditions, you should not do these poses. Instead, wait until later in the day, when you are ready for exercising and then bend backwards in a standing position (Fig. 4.21).

Position a in Fig. 4.9 is a left turn of the head, to follow position f in Fig. 4.8. Then bend the spine forward (Fig. 4.9). Positions b–e depict several stages of bending, with blue lines indicating the zones that may generate the encouragement signal. Position f usually generates such a signal in the shoulder joints, in the middle of the back, in the pelvic area, and in the knees and ankles.

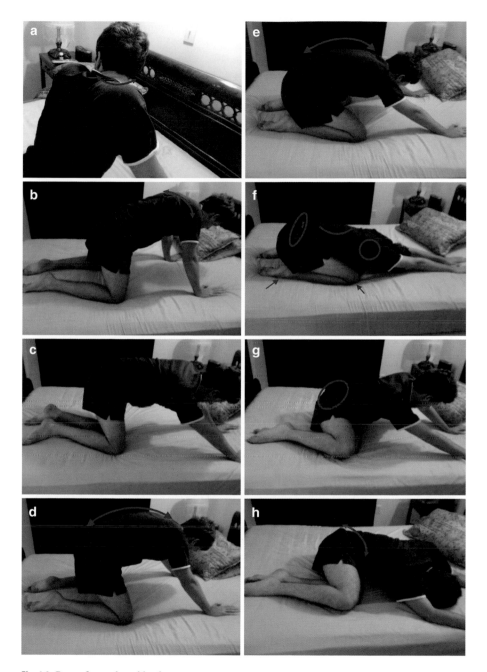

Fig. 4.9 Poses for neck and back

Positions g–h represent a group of twisting exercises. Twisting is a movement required in many locomotive routines like gait and running. It is also a tool for preventing falls due to unbalance. When we try to regain balance, compensatory movements occur quickly, and may lead to injuries if the skeleton is not prepared to the high loads associated with twisting of big masses like the trunk. Being in positions g–f is usually quite rewarding, both due to the high level of the pleasure signal, and the usefulness for the health of the skeleton.

4.5.5
Knee, Hip, and Pelvis Open Poses

We begin by lying on our backs (Fig. 4.10a). We gradually and slowly bend our knees (Fig. 4.10b–d).

To safely and painlessly cross our legs, we lift the bent knees, as shown in Fig. 4.10e, and slowly try to put them down on the bed. We do it with at least three stops in positions f–h. During these maneuvers, the pleasure sensation may be replaced by pain in some of the joints. We need to catch this from the first indication, and return to the pleasant zone.

These poses conclude the in-bed series.

4.6
Sanomechanical Day Series

We start the day series by laying supine like in Fig. 4.10a, but on a firm surface. The reason for this position is that between the moment when we stepped out of bed in the morning, and the time we allocate for the day's session, our skeleton and whole body has already accepted a lot of stresses and loads. Laying on a firm surface will relieve the joints from the compression caused by gravity acting down, and the ground reaction acting up.

Laying on a firm surface turns on the mechanism of passive stretching and straightening of the skeleton curves, as was explained in Sect. 4.3, and demonstrated in Figs. 4.1 and 4.2. Therefore, laying on a firm surface for a while is an excellent exercise on its own.

4.6.1
Knee, Hip, and Pelvis Open Pose – 2

The pose in Fig. 4.11 targets the hip joints, knee joints, and pelvis. When performed in bed, this pose was described with several incremental positions in Sect. 5.5. These positions (Fig. 4.10a–h) can be replicated on a floor mat to reach the final pose (Fig. 4.11).

The knee, hip, and pelvis open pose, like other sanomechanical exercises, activates those degrees of freedom in the joints which are generally inactive. It abducts the leg in the hip joints, rotates knees, and plantarflexes the foot in both the ankle and metatarsal joints. All these movements are not required for routine daily activities, and the ability to perform them diminishes with age. The necessity for good working conditions for these degrees of freedom

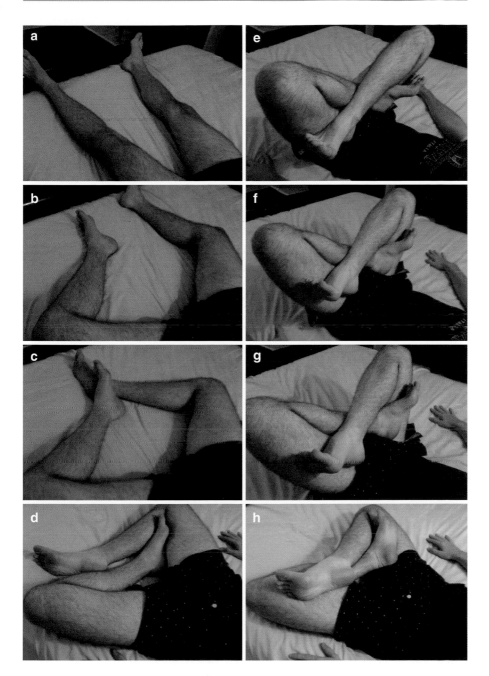

Fig. 4.10 Poses for knees, hips, and pelvis

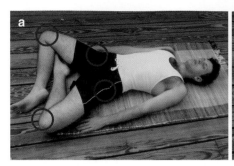
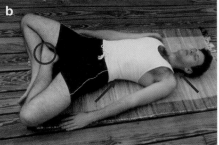

Fig. 4.11 Hip-knee-ankle pose. (**a**) *Blue circles* show areas of possible sensation of stretching. (**b**) When the feet are kept tighter, additional activation is sensed in ankle, lower back, and neck

occurs in challenging circumstances. It might be a walk on rough or slippery terrain, or when one stumbles, or when safety depends on more complex balancing than regular gait.

When entering the pose, you should stop at the very first position in which you feel a sensation of encouragement in any joint. Hold the pose for as long as this sensation is noticeable, and when it disappears, slowly continue.

If the knees do not initially touch the floor, they will sag under gravity once the muscles relax. Therefore, the uncomfortable sensation may come from the hips or groins before the knees reach the floor. In that case, begin the initial position with the knees less flexed. If you feel discomfort in any joint, go back until the discouragement signal is gone. The more you practice, the more joints will send positive signals simultaneously. It is good if you can enter the pose as shown in Fig. 4.11b without discomfort and with pleasure signals in several joints. Listen to your body signals carefully and respectfully. Remain in the pose for as long as it gives you pleasure. It might be several seconds or several minutes.

Remember, the goal of the exercise is not a "correct" body configuration or timing, but a dialog of your mind with your body. In that dialog, you allow your body to get exactly what it needs, according to the signals of the joint capsules and periosteum, which in return reduces pressures applied to the joints' cartilages, and increases skeletal flexibility.

4.6.2
Hip, Knee Rotation, Subtalar Pose

The knee joint formally has one degree of freedom: flexion/extension. However, the joint has some laxity, allowing for small rotation of the shin relative to the thigh. That mobility provides cushioning in fast maneuvers and abrupt stops in sports, and if that mobility is limited, the risk of injuries increases. Considering the significantly smaller range of motion in knee rotation compared to rotation in the subtalar joint (between the foot and the shin), the knee rotation is a backup for the latter – however, a very important one.

The position shown in Fig. 4.12, generates encouraging sensations in three joints: hip, knee, and subtalar. We begin by slowly flexing the knee and sweeping the heel outward. We stop as soon as the first positive signal appears. It could be in any of the

Fig. 4.12 Hip-Knee–Subtalar pose. *Blue circles* show possible areas of sensation of stretching

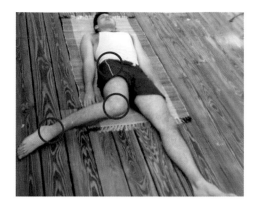

three joints involved. We will hold the pose until the sensation disappears, and will continue toward the final pose (Fig. 4.12).

The more you practice, the more acute the knee flexion angle will be at which the knee can remain on the ground. However, as with other sanomechanical exercises, your target is not a certain body configuration, but addressing the silent request of the body that you are evoking in a form of encouraging sensations.

4.6.3
Twisting Parallel Legs in Hip Joints

The initial position and gradual changing of the positions for this exercise were shown in the in-bed series (Fig. 4.7a–h). On a firm surface (Fig. 4.13), the encouraging signal (indicated by blue ovals) is perceived in the same zones as when this exercise was performed in bed. The level of sensation may be higher on the firm surface. However, if the surface is too firm, it might be difficult to lie for as long as in bed, up to the moment when the positive signal disappears, because of the high contact pressure on the hips and the pelvis on the floor mat.

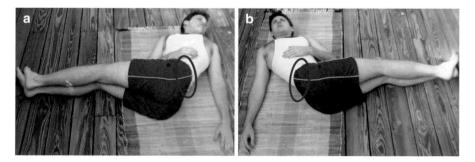

Fig. 4.13 Twisting parallel legs at the hip: (**a**) to the right; (**b**) to the left

The overall sensation on the floor mat is richer compared to the in-bed series, because the spine also straightens in the lumbar zone. Moreover, the vertebrae in the lumbar zone become involved in the twisting as well. The first signal may come from different joints, but should be immediately processed by you using the criterion of correctness. It is not a good idea to hold a position if one joint sends a positive signal, while another joint sends a negative signal in the form of pain. You should adjust the poses to eliminate pain, even if you feel that the encouragement sensation in some joint or joints is concurrently reduced.

4.6.4
Spine and Pelvis Poses – 2

In Fig. 4.14, we replicate the spine and pelvis poses previously described in the in-bed series (Sect. 4.5.4. and Fig. 4.8). The floor mat is the ideal surface and offers maximal benefits from the pose. We first look for a positive sensation in the lumbar zone of the spine. If your back is not very flexible in the lumbar zone, the positive signal comes rather quickly and your shoulders will be lower than shown in Fig. 4.14. For a positive sensation, it might not be necessary to extend the arms fully for support as in (a); as always, the arms should be flexed at the angle found using the criterion of correctness.

The less flexible your spine initially, the narrower the pleasant zone will be, and the quicker will be the passage into the zone of pain. In this case, you should hold the pose with the encouraging sensation for as long as possible, and move to the next position also as slowly as possible.

You can let your head droop as in Fig. 4.8d. You will need to begin to relax the neck muscles that support the head's position. As a result, the previous balance between the moment generated by these muscles and the force of gravity will be broken. The moment of the force of gravity will win, and the head will begin moving down, bringing the chin closer to the chest. Only now will you realize how heavy your head is. Be careful during the first angles of neck bending, and relax the neck muscles very slowly.

When exercising on a hard surface, you will better feel your pelvis's movement and the relative micro displacements of its bones. For visualization and autosuggestion, you may imagine how synovial liquid impregnates the tiny spaces between the pelvis's bones, its ligaments, and the periosteum.

The maximal encouraging sensation will be experienced when twisting the spine. Try seeing your heel by turning the head to the left (b) and right (c). It may not be possible at the beginning to actually see your heels. Forced attempts to achieve this goal may carry you to the pain zone, passing over the pleasure zone too quickly. You should not try to rush, since it may hurt you in a way you do not deserve.

Similar to the poses for the neck and back in Fig. 4.9f–h, we now proceed to flexing the lumbar zone and knees while extending the shoulders and feet (Fig. 4.15a).

This replicates the Yoga "child's pose" (Rawls 1966), in which both arms are extended backward, with the hands lying on the mat and the palms facing up. If you have practiced this pose before you now know how to make it *sanomechanical* for better results. As with all other poses you are familiar with, enter the pose and gradually progress with sanomechanical autosuggestion and the criterion of correctness.

Fig. 4.14 Bending the spine backward (**a**), followed by turning head to the left (**b**) and right (**c**)

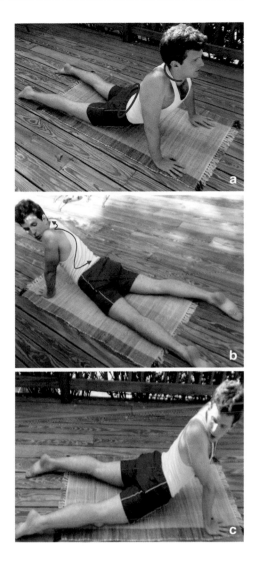

The position in Fig. 4.15a may be reached with several steps, each determined by the sensation of encouragement or discouragement (pain). After you are rewarded with a signal of pleasure in a new position, hold that position, until the signal disappears, and then when you pass to the next position you will be granted a new reward of pleasure. It is like walking through an enfilade where the door to the next room opens only after the door behind closes. In this passage, you will sense positive signals from the lower back, shoulders, knees, and ankle as marked in blue.

Subsequent positions b–d will give you positive signals in the pelvic area and in the spine. In the slow transition from one position to another, the initial angle λ_1 of the torso relative to the pelvis will be increasing ($\lambda_1 < \lambda_2,...$).

Fig. 4.15 Poses for back and pelvis. (**a**) Initial position; (**b**–**d**) Selected positions based on cycles of the encouraging sensation

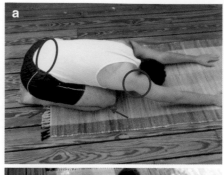

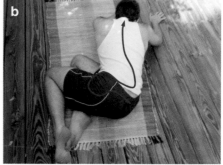

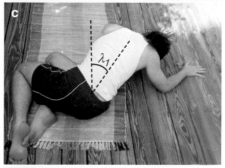

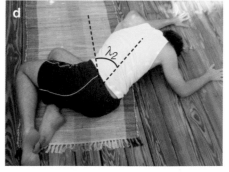

4.6.5
Foot, Ankle, and Toe Pose

The first pose in the standing position targets multiple degrees of freedom in the foot, ankle, and toes, which are less commonly utilized. The consequences of not using what is designed by nature are negative as usual. These joints, along with the joints of the fingers, are the first affected by arthritis and other similar disorders. The major reason for limited flexion in toes is shoe design, which allows for toe extension, but restricts their flexion.

What is the biomechanical rationale for toe flexion in gait? It provides the conditions for the body to be propelled forward without the foot's slipping backward. The coefficient of friction between the foot and the walking surface has to be no less than some lower threshold (Питкин 1985). The value of the foot's coefficient of friction is adjusted by the toes' stronger or weaker "grasp." Toes flex both when we walk barefoot and when we walk in shoes. A recording of the electrical activities of the toes' muscles confirms this (Fujita 1985; Morag and Cavanagh 1999).

An imprint of the toes' grasp on sand is shown in Fig. 4.16. Adjustment to the soil conditions and walking occurs automatically and every configuration of every toe is selected automatically as well (Fig. 4.16c). If the shoe's internal shape and volume do not allow for certain configurations of the flexed toes, it may lead to swelling, bunions, blisters, etc. The associated pain is a secondary source of even greater restrictions for the toes' articulation. What is important for us here is that restrictions on these articulations in the shoes leave many degrees of freedom unused.

The following pose (Fig. 4.17) will address the issue by providing the much needed articulations in the feet and toes. The pose has its roots in the folk dance called *Lezginka* from the Caucasus region (Fig. 4.18), and classical ballet.

The difference is that in *Lezginka* and ballet the performer jumps and lands on the flexed toes, loading them tremendously. In our pose (Fig. 4.17), we position the upper surface of the toes on the floor mat with the full body weight on the opposite leg and foot. We then slowly add portions of the involved leg's weight for loading the bent toes. Each step is controlled by the criterion of correctness, meaning that no pain is allowed to be ignored or sustained.

The blue curve along the foot in Fig. 4.17 indicates zones of possible sensations of encouragement we need to seek, and to hold until they are attenuated. The exercise is very rewarding, probably because of the rarity of such bending in the foot in our daily routine.

4.6.6
Knee and Ankle Standing Pose

We continue exercising while standing by bending the knee and holding our plantarflexed foot in our hand (Fig. 4.19a).

One cannot overestimate the importance of good mobility in the knee for healthy locomotion. During the first half of the support period, when the foot is on the walking/running surface, the knee flexes about 15° at each step. This is when the knee is most loaded. If the rolling cartilage surfaces are not well maintained within the synovial capsules, these loads

Fig. 4.16 Natural flexion of toes during walking on sand. Formation of a deep impression under the toes is marked with *red arrows* (**a**–**d**)

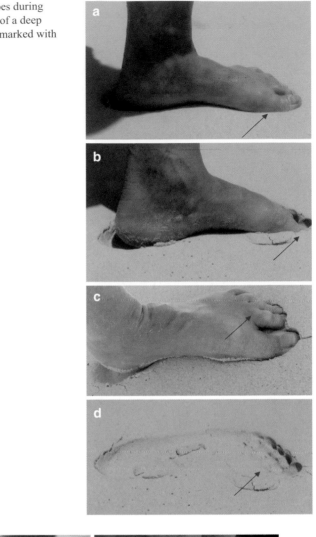

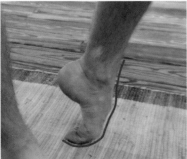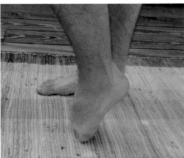

Fig. 4.17 Plantarflexion of the foot and flexion of toes

Fig. 4.18 Machmud Esambayev dancing "Lezginka" (With permission from RIA Novosti)

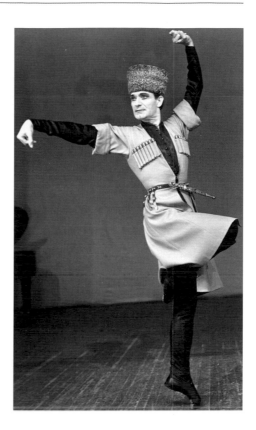

lead to cartilage damage and deterioration. With the theory of the hydraulic net involving neighboring joints (Chap. 1), we may assume further that a broken connectivity between the joints in the net would speed up the pathological changes in the knee cartilages.

To stop the unwanted development and make the knee joint better prepared for frequent extreme loads, the pose in Fig. 4.19, which looks like a typical *stretching* exercise, should be performed *sanomechanically*.

Zones with possible sensation of encouragement are indicated with blue circles in Fig. 4.19b. Since the two joints are under stress simultaneously, their signals may be different, and even when one of them sends a positive signal, the other may be in the pain zone.

- We need to "listen" carefully to what both joints are "saying" and adjust the angles in the knee and ankle in accordance with the criterion of correctness.
- Articulation within the knee angle's range of motion should be divided into three to four smaller ranges.
- The boundaries of these ranges are to be determined by first and subsequent zones of encouraging sensations.
- Autosuggestion prior to and during exercising has to be clear and conclusive: "My knee capsule is connected with the hydraulic net of the skeleton."

Fig. 4.19 Ankle and knee bending: (**a**) initial
position; (**b**) side view with the zones of
sensations of encouragement (*in blue*)

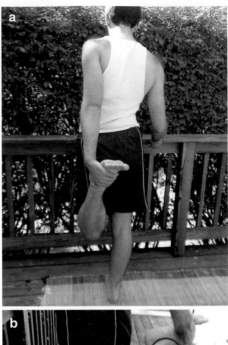

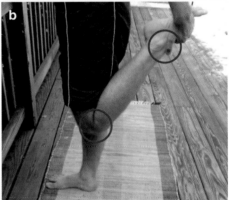

4.6.7
A Pose for Extension in Shoulder Joints and for Twisting the Torso

The shoulder joint has three degrees of freedom, but its movements in the horizontal plane[2]
are less in demand in our regular activities. We articulate more in the frontal[3] and sagittal[4]
planes. We should activate mobility in the horizontal plane first.

---

[2]*Horizontal plane* divides the body into superior and inferior parts
[3]*Frontal plane* is any vertical plane that divides the body into anterior and posterior parts
[4]*Sagittal plane* goes vertically from the top to the bottom of the body, dividing it into left and right
parts

We position the arms and twist the torso as shown in Fig. 4.20. The feet are perpendicular to the wall and should remain in that orientation for all cycles. We begin by twisting the torso to the left, trying to position the upper back parallel to the wall (Fig. 4.20a).

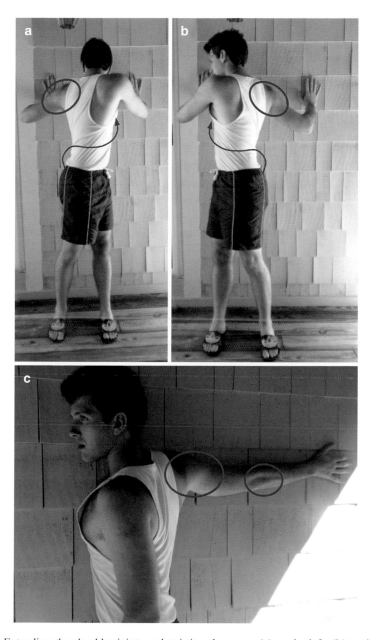

Fig. 4.20 Extending the shoulder joints and twisting the torso: (**a**) to the left; (**b**) to the right; (**c**) extension in elbow

Our first stop in the torso rotation occurs as soon as the first signal of encouragement appears in the spiral zone indicated with the blue line. When we hold the torso in this position, we are placing our hands on the wall and adjust their position in search of a positive signal from the left shoulder joint (indicated by the blue oval).

Once the positive signals from the spine and left shoulder disappear, we slide the hands to the left along the wall until the next pair of positive signals is generated.

After completing the cycle for the left twist of the torso, we repeat the same routine, this time twisting the torso to the right (Fig. 4.20b).

We may later add to this exercise an extension of the elbow joint (Fig. 4.20c) provided that we follow all the steps discussed above for the torso and shoulder poses.

4.6.8
Neck Bending

The purpose of neck bend exercises is to prepare the cervical part of your spine for the day's challenges, and/or to alleviate a discomfort you currently feel.

In Chap. 2, we discussed the neck bend in the frontal plane (Fig. 2.7). We used it as an example of a sanomechanical exercise because of its simplicity. Another reason was that neck bending should be one of the most frequent exercises you do and appreciate every day. Neck stiffness and pain are familiar to most adults who otherwise do not have any orthopedic or neurological problems.

In addition to bending in the frontal plane (to the left and right) (Figs. 2.7 and 4.21d), we will bend in the sagittal (Fig. 4.21a–b) and horizontal planes (Fig. 4.21c).

Please return to Sect. 2.4.2 and review the steps for doing the the exercises. It is critically important that all transitions from one encouraging position to another are performed very slowly and without any tension.

The autosuggestion for neck bending can be: "Because my vertebrae are soaked with synovial fluid, my neck is flexible like a snake."

4.6.9
Twisting Torso in Sitting Position

We continue twisting the torso in a sitting position on the floor mat. Intermediate positions (Fig. 4.22a–c) should be attained and held using the criterion of correctness. The exercise includes twisting the torso to the left with the left knee bent (e) and to the right with the right knee bent (f). Potential zones with encouraging signals are indicated in blue in Fig. 4.22f.

4.6.10
Roll on the Back

To complete the series and facilitate transition to regular daily activities, we will do a roll on the back exercise (Fig. 4.23a). We will swing back and forth several times, replicating the motions of an old fashioned ink-drier with a curved bottom on top of blotting paper.

Fig. 4.21 Neck bending: (**a**, **b**) sagittal plane; (**c**) horizontal plane; (**d**) frontal plane

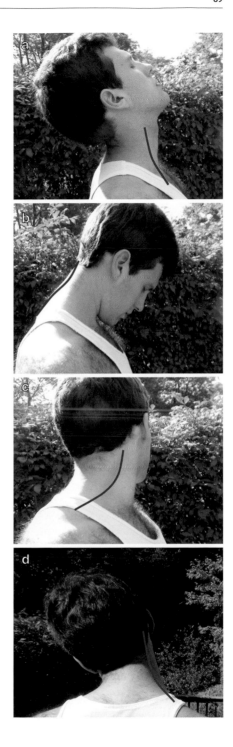

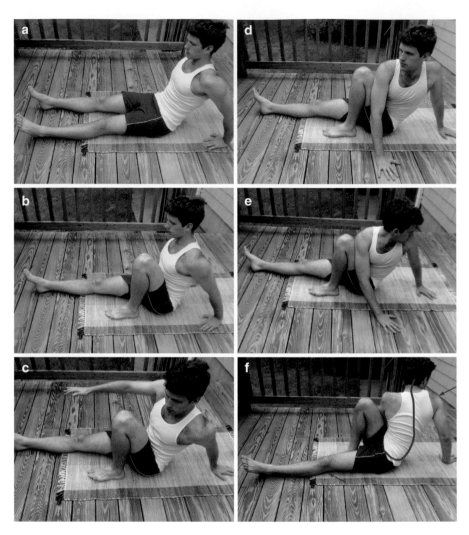

Fig. 4.22 Twisting torso in sitting position: (**a**) initial position; (**b**–**d**) twisting from right to left; (**f**) twisting from left to right

I like this analogy because the absorbing action of the blotting paper results from the effect of capillarity. It is capillarity which transports the ink from the writing surface to the blotting paper after the dryer rolls over the surface rolling. And it is capillarity too which transports synovial liquid along the spine after rolling on the mat.

The second phase of this exercise is to put both legs over the head in an attempt to reach the ground. It should be performed very carefully, as usual, with a slow search for intermediate positions that give encouragement. There is no way you should allow yourself to enter the pain zone (Fig. 2.6) in any part of your body.

Fig. 4.23 Rolling on the back (**a**), and touching the floor behind the head with the toes (**b**–**c**)

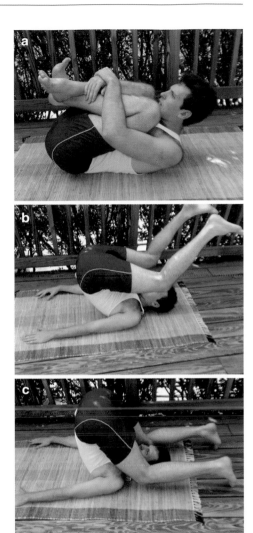

4.6.11
Completion of the Series

To complete the series and to maximize the effect of spreading the synovial liquid throughout the skeleton, we lie down on the back, catch a pleasant sensation from the final straightening of the lumbar zone of the spine, and say to ourselves: "My skeleton is fully soaked with the fluid."

4.7
Conclusion

There is no doubt that people who seriously and systematically practice yoga and other systems of perfecting body and mind are in better physical shape than the average population. So why, instead of creating new methods, shouldn't we just recommend yoga to everyone like William Atkinson, who introduced yoga to the Western World under the pseudonym Yogi Ramacharaka (Ramacharaka 1904, 1906, 1931)? Aren't sanomechanical exercises just a simplification of yoga, which teaches about escalating levels of physical and mental development and self-healing?

Sanomechanics is not meant to compete with yoga, nor to substitute it. Sanomechanics focuses on the mechanics of how the skeleton functions, and on the practical method of protecting the skeleton's structural integrity, flexibility, and overall health. Sanomechanics is based on a scientific concept explaining the sustainability of the human skeleton in the norm, and the reasons why its normal functioning may transform to pathology. The floating skeleton concept (Chap. 1) illuminates the causes for success or failure of the other systems of physical training.

To summarize:

- Success can be reached only if an effective restoration of hydraulic connectivity of synovial capsules is apparent.
- Further, sanomechanics shows how the hydraulic connectivity can be achieved.
- For an exercise to be sanomechanical, we need, in addition to the selected physical actions, to add autosuggestion, and a criterion for holding the poses in space and time.
- Finally, as we demonstrate in this book, sanomechanical exercises can be easily included in the real life of a busy person without especially dedicated hours for attending classes. It becomes a part of daily routine, which makes life safer and more enjoyable.

References

Fujita M (1985) Role of the metatarsophalangeal (MTP) joints of the foot in level walking. Nippon Seikeigeka Gakkai Zasshi 59(11):985–997

Morag E, Cavanagh PR (1999) Structural and functional predictors of regional peak pressures under the foot during walking. J Biomech 32(4):359–370

Nigg BM, Skarvan G, Frank CB, Yeadon MR (1990) Elongation and forces of ankle ligaments in a physiological range of motion. Foot Ankle 11(1):30–40

Perry J (1992) Gait Analysis: normal and pathological function. Slack, Inc., Thorofare

Pitkin MR (2010) Biomechanics of lower limb prosthetics. Springer, New York

Ramacharaka Y (1904) Hatha yoga. Yogi Publication Society, Chicago

Ramacharaka Y (1906) The science of psychic healing. Yogi Publication Society, Chicago

Ramacharaka Y (1931) A series of lessons in Raja yoga. Yogi Publication Society, Chicago

Rawls ES (1966) A handbook of yoga for modern living. Parker Pub. Co, West Nyack

Питкин МР (1985). Кинематические и динамические характеристики ходьбы в зависимости от фрикционных свойств опорной поверхности. Протезирование и протезостроение, сб. трудов вып. 73, М., ЦНИИПП: 98–102

About Forces and Moments in Locomotion

5

We will consider in this chapter the concepts of ballistics and resonance in gait. They will help us better appreciate how efficiently and economically human gait is organized. This information will give us additional reasons to pay more attention to our wondrous skeleton, which provides the perfect frame for the biomechanics of locomotion to function properly.

We will look into the ways of interpreting experimental data using theoretical models. We will look into the history and current techniques of biomechanical analysis of forces acting on the human body from outside and inside using gait analysis as an example. We will consider the assumptions and limitations of modeling the human body in motion; they help us interpret data better. The architecture of gait analysis and equipment for collecting kinematic and dynamic parameters are discussed. We will see why data provided by biomechanical analysis always require a fresh look for their interpretation.

Most of this chapter duplicates elements from our previous work (Pitkin 2010). Appearing only here are velocity and acceleration calculations for marker coordinates that are used in modeling a moving body by a stick figure, in addition to instructions for processing those coordinates.

5.1
Biomechanical Investigations of Gait

The current terms *motion analysis* and *gait analysis* relate to specialized hardware and software for collecting, processing, and analyzing kinematic and dynamic parameters of locomotion. We will consider here the structure of this methodology, its capability, and limitations.

Before the development of computerized motion analysis systems like Peak, Vicon, and others (Hirsch 2000), computation of joint angles, forces, and moments required significant efforts and were very time-consuming. The French astronomer Pierre Janssen may have suggested the use of cinematography in investigating locomotion; but it was first used scientifically by Etienne Marey (1830–1904), who also correlated ground reaction forces with movement, and pioneered modern motion analysis. Marey used one camera with a device that recorded movements on one photographic plate. In his studies of the human in motion, subjects wore black suits with metal strips or white lines (Fig. 5.1a), and they passed in front of black backdrops. Exposures of the photographic plate were made at a specified frequency, so the time intervals between consecutive images of the stick figures

M.R. Pitkin, *Biomechanics for Life*,
DOI: 10.1007/978-3-642-17177-2_5, © Springer-Verlag Berlin Heidelberg 2011

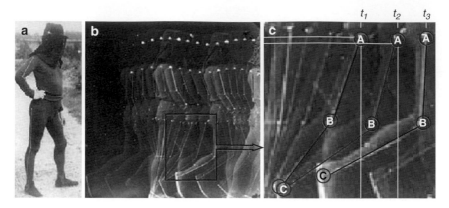

Fig. 5.1 (**a**) Marey's "Motion Capture" suite; (**b**) multiple images on the same photographic plate; (**c**) segments AB and BC at three consecutive times t_1, t_2, t_3 from the magnified area marked in (**b**)

were known (Fig. 5.1b). Coordinates of the markers from cinematography served as the input for the mathematical model of a poly-linker which simulated a human body.

One advantage of Marey's technique was the ability to calculate angles in joints versus time reasonably accurately. However, his breakthrough achievement was the practical way of computing accelerations of body segments, which opened the era of analysis of motion dynamics.

With Marey's images (Fig. 5.1b), let us consider how the stick model can be built analytically, and how accelerations of the markers can be computed using the formulas of analytic geometry (Spiegel and Liu 2001). The segments AB and BC at three consecutive times t_1, t_2, t_3 are taken from the area marked in Fig. 5.1b, and displayed with magnification in Fig. 5.1c. The first step is to measure the x, y coordinates of the points A, B, C and to develop the equations of the lines AB and BC for the times t_1, t_2, and t_3 (Fig. 5.2). The line through A(t_1) and B(t_1) is

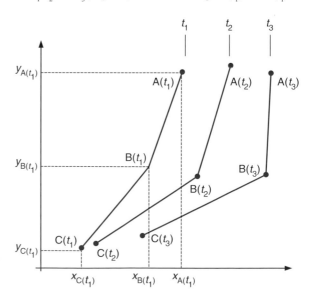

Fig. 5.2 The segments AB and BC at three consecutive times are taken from the area marked in Fig. 5.1b, and displayed with magnification in Fig. 5.1c

$$(x_{B(t_1)} - x_{A(t_1)}) \cdot (y - y_{A(t_1)}) = (y_{B(t_1)} - y_{A(t_1)}) \cdot (x - x_{A(t_1)}) \tag{5.1}$$

where $(x_{A(t_1)}, y_{A(t_1)})$ and $(x_{B(t_1)}, y_{B(t_1)})$ are the coordinates of $A(t_1)$ and $B(t_1)$, measured on the photo frame.

The line through $B(t_1)$ and $C(t_1)$ is:

$$(x_{C(t_1)} - x_{B(t_1)}) \cdot (y - y_{B(t_1)}) = (y_{C(t_1)} - y_{B(t_1)}) \cdot (x - x_{B(t_1)}) \tag{5.2}$$

Equations 5.1 and 5.2 are usually built into the software of contemporary computerized motion analysis systems that draw stick figures on a computer screen and perform further calculations.

To develop equations for calculating velocities and accelerations of the markers, we need to follow their movements in the x-t and y-t planes.

By definition, velocity is the slope of the line tangent to a point's trajectory. Thus,

$$
v_{y_{A(t_1)}} = \tan \beta_1 = \frac{y_{A(t_2)} - y_{A(t_1)}}{t_2 - t_1}
$$
$$
v_{y_{A(t_2)}} = \tan \beta_2 = \frac{y_{A(t_3)} - y_{A(t_2)}}{t_3 - t_2} \tag{5.3}
$$

Similarly, we get the x components of point A's velocities:

$$
v_{x_{A(t_1)}} = \frac{x_{A(t_2)} - x_{A(t_1)}}{t_2 - t_1}
$$
$$
v_{x_{A(t_2)}} = \frac{x_{A(t_3)} - x_{A(t_2)}}{t_3 - t_2} \tag{5.4}
$$

Since acceleration is defined as the slope of the line tangent to the velocity curve, the x, y components of point A's acceleration will be: $a_{x_{A(t_1)}} = \dfrac{v_{x_{A(t_2)}} - v_{x_{A(t_1)}}}{t_2 - t_1}$, and $a_{y_{A(t_1)}} = \dfrac{v_{y_{A(t_2)}} - v_{y_{A(t_1)}}}{t_2 - t_1}$, yielding the modulus of point A's acceleration at t_1 as

$$a_{A(t_1)} = \sqrt{\left(a_{x_{A(t_1)}}\right)^2 + \left(a_{y_{A(t_1)}}\right)^2} \tag{5.5}$$

Since Marey's technique allows us to compute accelerations of points that define the moving body's segments, it also allows us to use Newton's second law for translational and rotational movement. The law says that the acceleration $\overline{a}$ of the particle is proportional to the resultant force $\overline{F}$ acting on it and goes in the direction of that force:

$$m\overline{a} = \overline{F} \tag{5.6}$$

where m is the particle's mass.

When formulating Newton's second law for rotational movement, one needs to think not about force, but about the moment $\overline{M}$ as the source of angular acceleration $\overline{w}$, and about the *moment of inertia* instead of the mass of the particle. Application of Marey's routine for both translational and rotational motion yields both linear and angular accelerations of the body segments. As a result, forces and moments acting on the segments can be computed. When accelerations are known, the task of determining the forces and moments, as in our case (see Eq. 5.6), is called the *inverse problem of mechanics*.

The mathematical models of computerized motion analysis systems depend on the number of links in the poly-linker model, and on the conventions regarding their connection with each other. The models also include a stereometric transformation of the 2-D coordinates captured by the video camera frames into 3-D data. In addition, several assumptions have to be made about the geometry of mass. In most algorithms, free-body diagrams are built and calculation of forces and moments begins from the bottom up for every segment, starting with the foot (Meglan and Todd 1994). The resultant force $\overline{F}_r$ applied to the joint can be determined from the equation

$$\overline{F}_r = m\overline{a} - m\overline{g} - \sum_{i=1}^{n_j} \overline{F}_{ij} - \sum_{i=1}^{n_e} \overline{F}_{ei} \tag{5.7}$$

where m is the mass of the segment; $\overline{g}$ – acceleration due to gravity; $\overline{a}$ – acceleration of translation of the segment; $\overline{F}_{ij}$ – forces acting on the segment from n_j joints connected to this joint; $\overline{F}_{ei}$ – external forces applied to the segment. The resultant moment $\overline{M}_r$ acting on the segment is determined from Eq. 5.8:

$$\overline{M}_r = \overline{J} - \sum_{i=1}^{n_j} \overline{M}_{ji} - \sum_{i=1}^{n_j} \overline{p}_{ji} \times \overline{F}_{ji} - \sum_{i=1}^{n_e} \overline{M}_{ei} - \sum_{i=1}^{n_j} \overline{p}_{ei} \times \overline{F}_{ei} - \overline{p}_r \times \overline{F}_r \tag{5.8}$$

where the components of the vector

$$J = \left\{ \begin{matrix} I_{xx}\alpha_x + (I_{zz} - I_{yy})\omega_y\omega_z \\ I_{yy}\alpha_y + (I_{xx} - I_{zz})\omega_x\omega_z \\ I_{zz}\alpha_z + (I_{xx} - I_{yy})\omega_x\omega_y \end{matrix} \right\}$$

are formed by the segment's angular velocities, angular accelerations, and the components of the main moment of inertia (I_{xx}, I_{yy}, I_{zz}); $\overline{M}_{ji}$ is the moment applied to the joints connected to this segment; $\overline{M}_{ei}$ – moment acting on the segment from the outside; the vector products $\overline{p}_{ji} \times \overline{F}_{ji}$ are the moments applied to the joints; and the vectors $\overline{p}_{ji}$ describe the position of the joints in a coordinate system attached to the segment (Meglan and Todd 1994).

5.2
Modeling the Human Body for Motion Analysis and Related Equipment

Computerized motion analysis systems include a software package for customizing the model of the moving object under investigation. The moving object can either be a body part or a man-device system. A "device" can be a shoe, clothes, athletic equipment, or other pieces of the environment. Every such model requires a specific placement of the markers on the subject's body and on the device. There are also standardized schematics for the markers' placement, which decrease the time of the trial, and also allow for a more reliable comparison of results from different trials and different laboratories.

Systematically following the Marey method of representing the human body with a stick figure has led to a series of conventions about the number of markers and their positioning on a subject. The most popular is a schematic developed at the Helen Hayes Hospital, West Haverstraw, New York (Kadaba et al. 1989; 1990) (Fig. 5.3).

To customize the model for a specific subject, his/her anthropomorphic parameters (body mass, height, length of arms, legs, etc.) have to be added to the list of the averaged statistical data (McCronville et al. 1980).

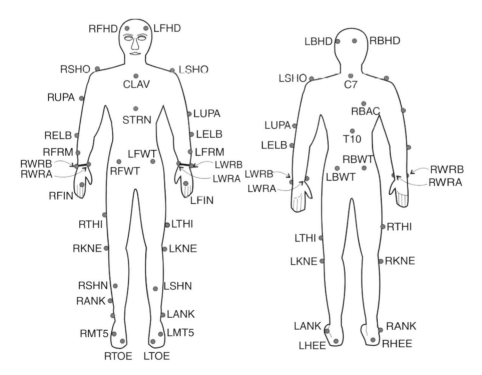

Fig. 5.3 Standard full body marker set (Adopted with permission from Vicon Motion Systems, Inc., Centennial, CO)

Equipment of the biomechanical laboratory may include among other components:

1. Video-based motion analysis system(s)
2. Force plate(s)
3. Pressure measurement system(s)
4. Instrumentation for EMG

Video cameras are attached to the walls or a ceiling, and the force plates are mounted inside the walkway. Video cameras capture images with a frequency in the range of 50–500 Hz; the computerized procedure allows the 3-D coordinates of the reflective markers to be calculated on a time scale. Using a body model selected by the researcher, the motion analysis system calculates joint angles, velocities, accelerations, temporal data, and other kinematic characteristics.

The force plate design is similar to piezoelectric or tensometric scales. Their prototype is the force plate introduced by Elftman (1938). The signal from the force plates is synchronized with the video camera images and satisfies Eqs. 5.7 and 5.8 (Antonsson and Mann 1985; Gillespie and Dickey 2003).

In force measurement, Kistler[1] sensors use the piezoelectric effect directly. The quartz sensor element generates a measurement signal proportional to the force applied. In a slightly modified form, torque or strain can also be measured directly (Rossi et al. 1995).

If a spatial force is applied in an unknown direction, only a three-component sensor is capable of detecting the total force simultaneously. This sensor captures the three orthogonal components F_x, F_y, and F_z. For this type of measurement, the piezoelectric sensor is preferable. Special sensors, similar in form to load washers, are used for measuring torque. The sensor measures the moment vector parallel to its own axis. The value of the torque is always measured relative to the origin of the coordinate system. The ability to measure the components of the ground reaction vector and its moment relative to all three coordinate axes makes force plates a necessary part of the equipment of a gait laboratory (Kerrigan et al. 1998).

Portable force plates with built-in 9286AA amps can be mounted within a walkway, which is installed on a regular floor. Kistler force plates can be integrated with almost any motion analysis system used in a biomechanics laboratory. If used independently, Kistler force plates should be operated with the *BioWare* data acquisition and analysis software package for research.

In combination with data from force plates, the motion analysis system calculates ground reactions, forces, and moments in joints.

5.3
Architecture of Computerized Gait Analysis

The Motion Capture industry has made extensive advances since the early days of digitizing video data. Today, 3-D data is available in real time and can be used in a wide range of applications. A schematic of the architecture of the data collection and analysis is shown in Fig. 5.4.

---

[1]Kistler Instrument Corp, Amherst, NY

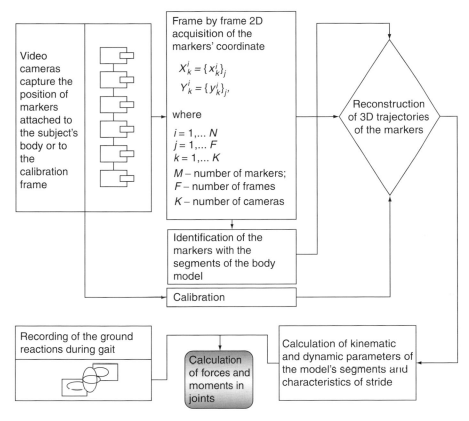

Fig. 5.4 Schematic of computerized gait analysis. Input – video signal and ground reactions. Output – kinematic and dynamic parameters of gait (Pitkin 2010)

The subject comes into a laboratory and has some basic physical measurements taken before the markers are placed on the person in the appropriate locations to conform to the testing protocol for that day. A static trial is captured, and some additional information is recorded by the software. The person then goes through the dynamic trials that were selected by the managing group or physician, and kinematic and kinetic data are collected. The relevant 3-D coordinate data and data from the force plates, EMG, or other equipment can all be seen on the screen instantaneously as the subject moves in the capture space. The data are collected on the computer and processed in a matter of seconds. A report with all the results of the test can be made available a few minutes after the data are collected (months of manual computational work were required at the beginning of the motion analysis era). A color video of the subject can also be shown alongside the 3-D workspace with a rendered skeleton or other mesh. The complete set of kinematic and kinetic variables is available on graphs.

Interpretation of the results of computerized gait analysis requires clinical experience, and a clear understanding of the method's limitations (Zajac et al. 2003; Simon 2004; Pitkin 2009). While the video cameras have 0.1-mm precision in determining the markers'

Fig. 5.5 Example of a bony model with a set of muscles from the video component of a report generated by the Vicon Motion Analysis System (New England Sinai Hospital Center for Human Performance, Stoughton, MA)

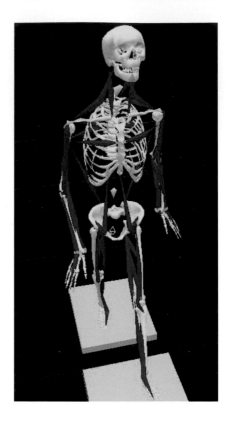

position within the 2-D frame, measurement errors are multiplied if marker placement is not consistent. To increase the reliability of the conclusions, it is better to analyze data collected in the same laboratory. The reliability is improved when data are collected from the same subject whose markers remain unchanged during all trials in the session.

Standardized report templates (Fig. 5.5) which are part of a system software package may contain superfluous information, not relevant to the specifics of a particular study. At the same time, the templates may not display data which are important for the study. Therefore, the format of the report has to be evaluated along with the study design and before the study begins.

5.4
Ballistic Synergy in Normal Gait

We consider gait as a cyclic process that maximally harnesses gravity by coordinated changes of the body's configuration. The body's configuration changes during the gait cycle when the joint's mobility changes from free to limited at a certain degree, with total locking being the extreme case. Any deviations from the coordinated sequence of configuration changes result in an increase of compensatory movements.

Synergic movements in gait require minimal control, since only a portion of all degrees of freedom of the body has to be used (Bernstein 1967). Aristotle and Plato promulgated the idea that the main attributes of biped gate are the body's periodic free and interrupted falls, and the periodic recuperation of the vertical coordinate of the body's center of mass. The Weber brothers revived this idea in the middle of nineteenth century (Weber and Weber 1991/1836). They combined the idea about well-organized falls with the notion of proper utilization of gravity and ground reactions, which laid the basis for the development of contemporary ballistic models of gait and the construction of walking machines (Collins et al. 2005).

Among many approaches in building walking biped machines, only the approach of "ballistic synergy" seems to be promising. It simplifies control and lowers the demand for power supplies (Mochon and McMahon 1979; McGeer 1990; Goswami et al. 1996; Dankowicz et al. 2001), as compared to robots all of whose degrees of freedom in motion are controlled during the entire gait cycle (Miura and Shimoyama 1984; Yamaguchi et al. 1996).

The consideration of the ballistic elements of gait was traditionally limited to the swing phase, when the load on the leg is minimal. For the stance phase, when the loads are at their maximum, the advantages of ballistic representation of gait were first considered in our works on ankle and knee joints in the norm (Pitkin 1975; Питкин 1975, 1977, 1980, 1985; Pitkin 1984). We analyzed the unique function of the foot plantar flexors. That unique function is to slow down the dorsiflexion (see Fig. 3.15 for definition) and eventually terminate it. As a result, angular velocity in the ankle changes its sign when plantarflexion starts, the heel lifts, and rotation passes from the ankle to the metatarsal joint. We attributed these events to the ballistic synergy of normal gait (Pitkin 1997; Pitkin 2006a, b).

5.4.1
Generation of the Propulsive "Push-off"

The role of the anatomical foot and ankle in generation of propulsion was investigated in many laboratories both for purely scientific reasons and in response to rehabilitation needs. Since 1939, when they became available, force plate data have provided major objective input to understanding how the foot functions. Analyzing the energy transfer during the stride, Elftman first presented the classic bimodal curve of the vertical ground reaction force (Elftman 1939). Elftman concluded that during the final stage of the stance period, the rest of the body received energy from the leg. That consideration became the foundation for the theory of the push-off as a major source for body propulsion.

More specifically, the theory went that the ankle plantar flexors (*m. gastrocnemius* and *m. soleus*) play a major role in body propulsion during the second peak of the ground reaction force. Support for the theory comes from the observation that the maximal EMG activity of *m. gastrocnemius* and *m. soleus* at push-off coincides with an increase in the total mechanical energy of the body. Also, the high power generated in the ankle exceeds that in the knee and hip joints (Sutherland 1966; Морейнис et al. 1971; Winter 1979; Sutherland et al. 1980a; Hof et al. 1983; Perry 1992; Rab 1994; Kepple et al. 1997). In a Winter study (Winter 1983) of normal gait in 15 subjects, it was demonstrated that ankle power is three times greater than power in the knee and hip joints.

In contrast to the "push-off" propulsion theory, there were studies which did not attribute propulsion to the ankle (Saunders et al. 1953; May and Davis 1974; Breakey 1976; Богданов and Гурфинкель 1976; Skinner and Effeney 1985; Perry 1992; Lehmann et al. 1993; Czerniecki 1996; Kirtley 2005). One of the reasons is clinical practice, with examples of satisfactory compensation for different types of pathology, including amputation. A convincing case was presented by Murray in a gait study of a woman whose *m. gastrocnemius* and *m. soleus* were surgically removed (Murray et al. 1978). Biomechanical analysis revealed compensatory excursion of the pelvis, prolonged activity of quadriceps, and greater angle of dorsiflexion in the involved leg. Nevertheless, her gait pattern remained almost intact and symmetric, which wouldn't be possible if the propulsion were generated solely by foot flexors.

Some researchers have characterized the ankle plantar flexors as accelerators that facilitate the movement of the leg into the swing phase (Dillingham et al. 1992; Meinders et al. 1998; Pitkin 2009). The study by Meinders et al., showed that during push-off, 23.1 Joules (J) of energy were generated, primarily by the ankle plantar flexors, but only 4.2 J of this energy was transferred to the trunk. The authors concluded that the ankle plantar flexor's work is primarily used to accelerate the leg into the swing phase. They also suggested that the existing controversy on the role of the foot plantarflexion results from the multiple roles the foot plays in human locomotion.

The continuing dispute about the generation of body propulsion and the contribution of body segments to this process is not only of academic interest. It is important for engineering and also for physical education and rehabilitation. Understanding the involvement of certain muscle groups in ballistic propulsion has direct impact on selecting the exercises for effectively loading the targeted muscles.

5.4.2
Regular and Intentional Push-off

To develop compelling arguments in favor or against the push-off propulsion theory, we designed and conducted two gait studies, followed by a computer simulation (Pitkin 2009). One gait study was associated with normal, level (regular) gait. The other tested the gait with intentional exaggerated push-off by the trailing leg. Compared to regular gait, the intentional push-off gait generated greater power in the ankle, and the knee in the trailing leg was locked. The subjects were not instructed to lock their knees – the locking occurred unintentionally.

In order to separate the effects of the foot's push-off and the stance knee's extension on propelling the body's center of mass, a computer simulation of foot propulsion was run. Besides the model of regular gait, we developed two models of propelling the body from the initial static stage. The first model had the unlocked knee as in the regular gait model. The second had the knee joint locked. By running the simulation, we found regular body propulsion only in the model with the locked knee. The model with the unlocked knee produced knee flexion seen in the pre-swing of regular gait without propelling the body's center of mass. Let us look closer at this study and discuss its outcomes.

5.4.2.1
Regular Push-off

Kinematic and dynamic gait analysis data in one healthy male subject were obtained with the VICON Motion Analysis System, at the Center for Human Performance of New England Sinai Hospital, Stoughton, MA. The subject was instructed to walk at a self-selected speed in his regular style. Data on angles, moments, and power in the ankle, knee, and hip joints were normalized for the subject's weight and duration of stride time (stance time + swing phase is 100%) (Fig. 5.6).

The vertical line defines the time between the stance and swing phases, and is approximately 60% of the stride time. Power in the ankle joint reaches its maximum at the end of the stance phase (Fig. 5.6a). The ankle's power peak correlates to a decrease in dorsiflexion and transfer to plantarflexion. The fact that the power maximum coincides with the

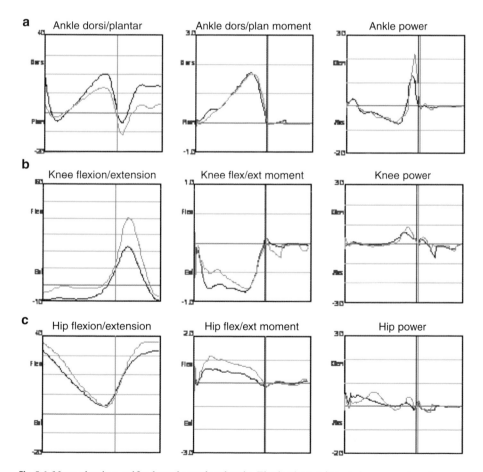

Fig. 5.6 Normal gait at self-selected speed and style. Flexion/extension angle, moment, and power in joints of left (*red*) and right (*green*) leg: (**a**) ankle; (**b**) knee; (**c**) hip (Pitkin 2010)

beginning of foot plantarflexion may be considered to be an indication that the ankle is the generator of the propulsion push-off. However, it can be interpreted this way only if taken independently from data on knee performance. If we add the performance of the knee joint to our consideration, we come to another result. Indeed, flexion in the knee begins simultaneously with the foot plantarflexion and even slightly prior to plantarflexion. Since the knee yields, it absorbs the push-off impulse from the foot. Consequently, it cannot transfer that impulse to the body's center of mass, as opposed to the traditional belief (Hof et al. 1983). Yielding of the knee when the foot is in plantarflexion can explain the low rate (a 25%) of transfer of power generated by the foot flexors to the trunk (Meinders et al. 1998).

A question arises: if the foot plantarflexion (push-off) in the trailing leg does not generate the propulsion of the body, then how is the propulsion generated? We compared the moments in the knee and hip joints along with the vertical component of ground reaction. The comparison reveals that the peaks of both moments occur simultaneously at 10–15% of stride, coinciding with the first maximum of the vertical component of the ground reaction. That synchronous extension in the knee and the hip joints of the forward leg (Fig. 5.6b, c) provides the upward acceleration of the center of mass and is the major source of the propulsion as we suggested earlier (Pitkin 1975), and as it has been observed by other researchers (Riley et al. 2001).

5.4.2.2
Intentional Push-off

The second gait experiment was conducted to demonstrate that the foot and ankle joint can primarily generate real body propulsion, if such a task is specifically requested. The same subject whose normal gait data are shown in Fig. 5.6, was instructed to walk by generating the intentional push-off with the feeling of his foot as the major actuator for propulsion of the body (Fig. 5.7). The subject reported an additional load to his calf muscles and additional pressure on the forefoot sole.

During the course of this type of gait, the power maximum in the ankle (Fig. 5.7a) was approximately 1.5 times greater than in normal regular gait (Fig. 5.6a), and the timing of that maximum came noticeably earlier than in normal regular gait. Deceleration and termination of the dorsiflexion in ankle and the switch to plantarflexion also occur noticeably earlier than in normal regular gait. The amplitude of the ankle angle and amplitude of the ankle moment are approximately 25% higher.

The increases in ankle angle, moment, and power indicate that the subject was able to generate a stronger push-off from the foot. Could one conclude that this push-off was indeed body propulsion? We believe that the answer should be in the affirmative due to the following arguments.

- The active flexion of the foot correlated with the locking of the knee joint in the extended position (Fig. 5.7b).
- That locking was produced by a moment whose value is noticeably higher than in regular gait (Fig. 5.6b).
- Therefore, the propulsive impulse was not cushioned in the knee, but was transferred to the body's center of mass.

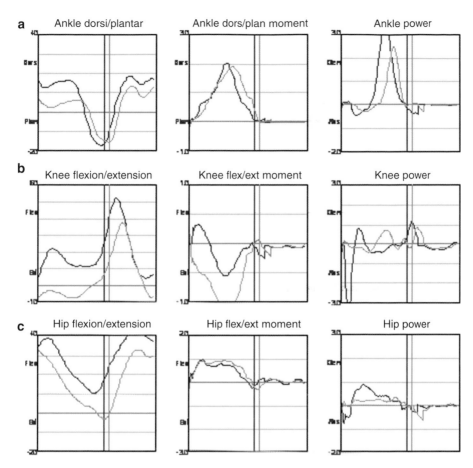

Fig. 5.7 Gait with a task of intentional aggravated push-off action of the foot. Flexion/extension angle, moment, and power in joints of left (*red*) and right (*green*) leg: (**a**) ankle; (**b**) knee; (**c**) hip (Pitkin 2010)

5.4.3
Computer Simulation of Regular and Intentional Gait

A walking style which we call here normal or regular belongs to the category of well automated locomotor actions. It doesn't require constant attention or control over the exact placement of the feet, nor over the sequence in which the muscles should be activated or relaxed. The shortest characterization of regular gait is that there is no need to think about it. That is how soldiers march, covering long distances with minimal energy expenditure. The elusive simplicity of regular gait shadows the mechanisms of coordination not yet well understood (Bernstein 1967; Sutherland et al. 1980b).

In contrast to the energetically efficient regular normal gait, any deviations from the automotive algorithm are associated with higher energy expenditure. If gait deviations determine a new gait style, like in our experiment with the intentional push-off propulsion, extra time is required for specific learning (Abe et al. 2004).

Fig. 5.8 "Working Model" simulation of the regular gait "push-off" event. The foot plantarflexion coincides with propulsion of the body's center of mass. It coincides also with the beginning of the knee flexion in the trailing leg, indicating that the yielding leg cannot transfer the push-off impulse to the body's center of mass. Frames are shown at 0.05 s intervals. Extension knee moment in the forward leg is shown by a small spring (Pitkin 2010)

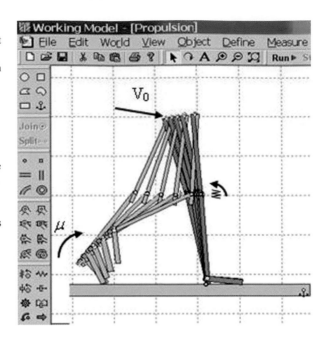

We will discuss a computer model of the propulsion in regular gait with the Working Model[2] software. The model (Fig. 5.8) consists of two legs, each having three links (foot, shin, and thigh). The torque μ in the ankle of the trailing leg simulates the foot plantarflexion. The center of mass has initial velocity V_0 acquired at the end of the swing phase of the forward leg. The knee in the forward leg has a passive rotational spring simulating the stance knee flexion/extension. Free rotation is allowed in the knee of the trailing leg, which provides ballistic flexion in the knee under gravity. Static moments of the limbs were taken to match the anthropomorphic data on the leg segments (McCronville et al. 1980). The model kinematics resemble the kinematics of normal walking with the center of mass moving forward and up after foot plantarflexion (Perry 1992). However, it remains not obvious, as in human gait, what the primary source of propulsion of the body's center of mass is. The uncertainty is caused by the simultaneous contribution of the torque in the ankle of the trailing leg, and the presence of the initial kinetic energy of the center of mass having velocity V_0. To resolve the controversy, we separated the action of the ankle torque and the center of mass's kinetic energy in the following two models.

The model shown in Fig. 5.9 differs from the model of regular gait propulsion by eliminating the initial velocity V_0 of the body's center of mass. All other model features are the same. The Working Model movie simulation begins with torque μ in the ankle of the trailing leg. It is seen from Fig. 5.9 that the trailing leg is flexing in the knee and going to the swing phase, similar to the regular gait model. Despite the foot's generating the same push-off moment, the position of the center of mass does not change. This indicates that the push-off action in the trailing leg cannot produce body propulsion when the torque is generated in the ankle and the foot is in plantarflexion.

---

[2]Design Simulation Technologies, Inc., Canton, MI 48187, USA

Fig. 5.9 "Working Model" simulation of the "push-off" event in static stage ($V_0=0$). The foot plantarflexion does not produce the propulsion of the body center of mass. The beginning of the knee flexion in the trailing leg occurs as in the model of the regular gait (Fig. 5.8). Frames are shown at 0.05 s intervals (Pitkin 2010)

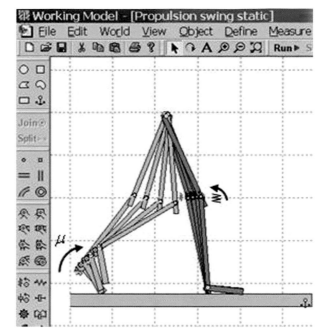

5.4.4
Simulation of Intentional Propulsion

The model of intentional propulsion Fig. 5.10 simulates the human trial with the task of predominantly using the torque in the ankle of the trailing leg. Its initial stage is static ($V_0 = 0$) as in the model in Fig. 5.8, but in addition, the knee in the trailing leg is locked. When the Working Model movie simulation begins, the trailing leg is transferring the impulse from the foot plantarflexion to the center of mass. As seen from Fig. 5.10, the position of the center of mass changes similarly to the model of regular gait Fig. 5.8.

Thus, we demonstrated that during regular gait foot plantarflexion does not substantially contribute to generating body propulsion. The main argument against the push-off propulsion theory is that the knee of the trailing leg flexes at the time of push-off. That flexing (yielding) of the knee joint prevents the push-off impulse from being transferred to the body's center of mass.

5.4.5
"Angle-Moment" Dependency in Ankle During Normal Gait

As we saw in the previous section, there are objectively registered differences between regular and exaggerated generation of the push-off. Let us try now to clarify what the foot and ankle are designed for if we don't attribute body propulsion to them. There are sufficient data on standing, walking, and running in the norm that confirm the coordinated alternation of free and limited mobility in joints (Sutherland 1966;

Fig. 5.10 "Working Model" simulation of the "push-off" event in static stage ($V_0=0$) with the locked knee in the trailing leg. The foot plantarflexion produces the propulsion of the body's center of mass similar to the model of regular gait (Pitkin 2010)

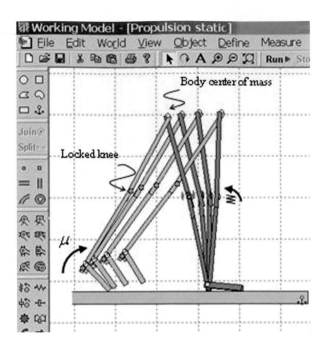

Winter 1979; Perry 1992). In the ankle, virtually free mobility occurs during the first two thirds of the dorsiflexion period, when the electric activity of the foot plantar flexors is very low. During the last third of the dorsiflexion period, the muscles' activity increases, and this correlates with the slowing down of dorsiflexion (Winter 1979; Mann et al. 1986).

Gait studies conducted at the Center for Human Performance of New England Sinai Hospital support our previous suggestion about the role of calf muscles in producing a moment in the ankle joint (Pitkin 1975; Pitkin 1977; Pitkin 1995), namely, that the major role of the plantar flexors is in braking dorsiflexion. Consequently, the foot's plantarflexion, which follows dorsiflexion, is the secondary assignment for these muscles.

The stance phase is divided into 7 consecutive phases, beginning with "heel-on" event 1 (Fig. 5.11). In the interval between events 2 and 3, the first plantarflexion is completed, and the foot's sole is in full contact with the walking surface. Dorsiflexion then begins, and continues until event 5 "heel-off." The heel lifts, and rotation is transferred from the ankle to the metatarsal joint (events 6–7). We will see further that this transfer utilizes inertia, and as such, is a component of ballistic gait synergy. The pattern of the moment's graph during the dorsiflexion period suggests very small resistance to dorsiflexion at the beginning of the period (2–3), a fast increase of the resistance prior to "heel-off" (4–5), and a fast drop during the second plantarflexion (7).

This sequence of events confirms our theory that the major role of the ankle moment is to slow down dorsiflexion, and to lock the ankle joint, but not to generate the body's propulsion. The "angle-moment" diagram is substantially nonlinear, with a slow rise and jump-like increase when the ankle joint has to be locked.

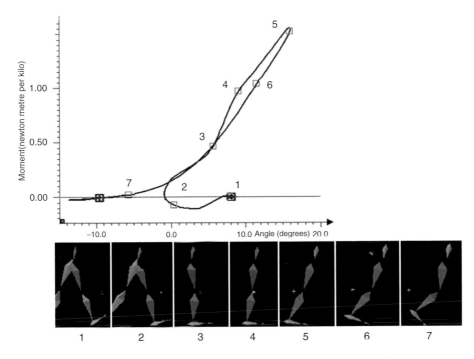

Fig. 5.11 Ankle moment as a function of the ankle angle in the norm. Events 1–7 correspond to consecutive phases of stance beginning with "heel-on" (Pitkin 2010)

5.4.6
Contribution of Knee to Ballistic Synergy

A specialist in physical medicine and rehabilitation has to have his/her own conceptual filter when analyzing published biomechanical data. That is especially true when dealing with patients with knee problems.

We will consider here the role of knee extension, which is antigravitational activity. As such, it has to require substantial external power from the surrounding muscles. However, a well-documented phenomenon is known about the surprisingly low electrical activity in the *m. quadriceps.* (Богданов and Гурфинкель 1976; Gage 1990; Rose and Gamble 1994; Laaksonen et al. 2006; Tseng et al. 2006). We say "surprisingly" regarding the low activity of these muscles during knee extension because before that period, the knee is flexing, and the activity of *m. quadriceps* is at its highest level. Therefore, the ability of the body to extend the knee without significant energy expenditure in the knee muscles merits investigation.

Traditionally, the activity of the knee extensors has been attributed to the resultant ground reaction vector, which becomes positioned anteriorly to the knee joint and generates a moment facilitating the knee's extension. At the end of the stance phase, the position of that vector becomes posterior relative to the knee joint, helping the knee flexion that is needed in the coming swing phase (Perry 1992).

We fully agree with this classic explanation, but believe that it reflects only one aspect of the energy efficiency of knee extension during stance. We suggest one more component of the knee extension phenomenon: an energy return after eccentric contraction of the muscles resisting the knee flexion during load acceptance (Saunders et al. 1953; Rab 1994).

We are going to discuss in more detail how propulsion is generated in normal gait using ballistics. From there, it will be clearer what we lose if our natural skeletal flexibility becomes reduced. With this understanding, the need for the sanomechanical approach to restoration of such a valuable feature of the body will be more substantive.

5.4.7
Generation of Propulsion in Norm and Consequences of Disruption of Ballistic Synergy in Gait

There is a well-known problem, given in most courses on mechanics, about calculating the floor reaction for a person standing inside an elevator which begins its way up or down. A solution is given by applying Newton's second law for a point with mass m, which moves along a vertical line. What is required from the student is correctly directing the vectors $\bar{a}$, of the body's acceleration from the elevator's floor, acceleration of the force of gravity $\bar{g}$ and floor reaction $\bar{N}$ in the equation

$$m\bar{a} = m\bar{g} + \bar{N}$$

Thus, if the coordinate axis is pointing up, the body's acceleration during accelerated lifting will be positive, and

$$ma = -mg + N.$$

Consequently,

$$N = mg + ma,$$

meaning that floor reaction will be greater than body weight at the value ma. Similarly, when the elevator begins going down

$$N = mg - ma,$$

meaning that the floor reaction is smaller than the body weight by ma.

That increase or decrease in ground reactions is recorded in normal gait when the body's center of mass (COM) accelerates up and down as a result of coordinated articulation in the hip, knee, and ankle joints. The phenomenon of inequality of the ground reaction and body weight is illustrated with a *Working Model* simulation (Fig. 5.12).

As shown in the left part of the simulation screen (Fig. 5.12), a rectangular block is moving down under gravity, as the body weight is higher than the force of initial resistance of the two springs, and moving up when the two springs are discharging. The graph above indicates the corresponding decrease and increase of the ground reaction F_y.

The right part of the screen shows a three-segment body model with ankle and knee joints, and the center of mass (COM) located at the upper segment. The ankle joint has "free-to-stop" mobility, and the knee joint has a rotational spring tuned for the body's

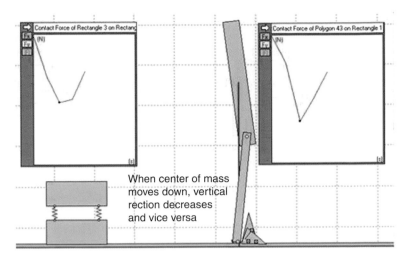

Fig. 5.12 Oscillation of vertical ground reaction depending on vertical movements of the center of mass (Pitkin 2010)

oscillation under the forces of gravity, spring resistive moment, and ground reaction. At the beginning of the simulation, the ground reaction is equal to the body weight. When the COM accelerates down, the ground reaction decreases and vice versa. It is important to note that the model has free mobility in the ankle and the option to stop, in order to limit it at a predetermined angle. If the ankle were immobilized, the model would not be in dynamic balance if the knee flexed.

Having illustrated here that the acceleration of the COM changes ground reactions, we can look at this phenomenon from another side: changes in ground reactions indicate that the COM is accelerating.

Let us see what we can say about accelerations of the COM by observing the typical graphs of the vertical component of the ground reactions (Fig. 5.13).

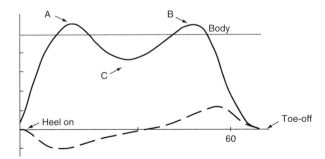

Fig. 5.13 Typical vertical (*solid line*) and anterior-posterior (*dashed line*) components of the ground reaction during stance in normal gait, normalized by body weight. Duration of stride (stance and swing phases) is 100%. A, B – peaks of vertical component; C – minimum of vertical component

The vertical reaction in normal gait usually has two peaks A and B whose values exceed body weight and a trough C whose value is lower than the body weight (Kadaba et al. 1989; Oberg et al. 1993). Based on our previous considerations, we may conclude that the COM of a subject is accelerated upward two times (before A and B), and downward also two times (between A and C, and after B). Since the upward acceleration of the COM is the indicator of antigravitational activity, both peaks have to be examined for their association with body propulsion.

Looking at the horizontal (anterior-posterior) ground reaction graph, we can see that the two peaks have different signs, where the negative sign is associated with backward direction and the positive – sign with forward direction. This reflects that during the first half of the stance phase the resultant vector of the ground reaction is oriented backward–upward, and, after the horizontal component changes its sign from minus to plus, is oriented forward–upward.

Analysis shows that the foot's "push off" occurs after the COM acceleration reaches its maximum (peak B), and that it coincides with knee flexion, thereby reducing the power transfer from the trailing leg to the COM. This allows us to conclude that the main contribution to body propulsion comes not from the foot, but from the hip joint and trunk's movement and the antigravitational flexion/extension in the knee.

The role of the foot's "push-off" and the knee's antigravitational flexion/extension in generating propulsion increases when we run, and both peaks A and B of the ground reaction merge in to a unimodal curve.

For people suffering from osteoarthritis, significant deviations from normal knee extension were found to be correlated negatively with physical activity (Watanabe et al. 2010), with some distinctions between the gait pattern in males and females. That means that the COM does not undergo the normal sequence of positive and negative accelerations. The disruption of normal ballistic synergy affects the function of stance knee flexion/extension and its coordination with adequate dorsiflexion in the ankle.

Therefore, a restoration of ballistic synergy has to be on the list of remedies addressing osteoarthritis and other musculoskeletal disorders. The first step in that direction should be restoration of natural flexibility of the skeleton in conjunction with corresponding control from the nervous system over the coordinated sequence of free and restricted mobility in each joint. Sanomechanics can be a practical way for achieving this goal.

5.5
Resonance and Anti-resonance

In this section, we will discuss some aspects of biomechanics of locomotion related to resonance and anti-resonance. These provide additional arguments for maintaining a healthy flexibility of the skeleton, which allows the body to effectively control our movements with maximal safety. Using normal gait and running as examples, we will show the rationale for considering tuning out of resonance to be a phenomenon at least as important as tuning into resonance. The latter is a traditional topic in biomechanical analysis, while anti-resonance activity in the human body has been investigated only recently (Pitkin 2008). We suggest a model of spectral optimization where the control vector consists of stiffnesses in joints. This approach bridges resonance and anti-resonance control with the problem of preventing falls. To effectively prevent falls and other disruption of normal locomotion, the skeleton has to function within its anatomical ranges of motion, providing biomechanical conditions for free articulation when it is required by the biomechanical control system. Deeper familiarity with biomechanics of locomotion may persuade our *super ego* to give higher priorities to the *id* needs of our skeleton, before it will demand it undeniably through pain and suffering.

5.5.1
Concept of Resonance in Biomechanics of Human Locomotion

Any movement in any single joint is of rotational type. As a consequence, a point marked on the segment will generate a piece of an arc, rather than a straight line. As Aristotle (384 BC–322 BC) noticed, if any point of a human leg or arm moves along a straight line, at least two joints must be involved (Aristotle 1934, 1981). Coordination of simultaneous movements in even two joints is a task that may require training. It certainly does require training to draw a perfectly straight line, or to generate perfect trajectories specific to sports played at a high level. Besides the involvement of at least two joints, there is one more similarity between drawing a line and of a professional athlete's motion. To generate the needed trajectory for an endpoint of a limb or a device, the rotations in each of the involved joints should neither be too slow nor too fast and should be as ballistic as possible. These *quantum satis* rotations are the oscillations at the so-called natural frequency, specific to each of the limb segments. The natural frequency of a segment is determined by the distribution of its mass (*moment of inertia*). If the driving rotational moment is consistently applied with the natural frequency, the amplitude of oscillation reaches its maximum.

The phenomenon is called *resonance* and can be examined by pushing a mathematical pendulum consisting of a weightless rod of length l_1 pivoted without friction about the hinge at its upper end and a bob of mass m_1 located at its lower end. We can learn from experimenting with the frequency of pushing impulses that when the pendulum is pushed with a certain frequency, it will swing higher and higher, and the pushes required are relatively small. We can, in this way, experimentally find the pendulum's natural frequency. Theory says that the natural frequency v_1 for an ideal pendulum does not depend on its mass and is determined only by its length, as in Eq. 5.9:

$$v_1 = \frac{1}{2\pi}\sqrt{\frac{g}{l_1}} \qquad (5.9)$$

Qualitatively, Eq. 5.9 teaches that the longer the pendulum's rod, the lower its natural frequency will be, and vice versa (Rosenberg 1991). A practical way to learn about the natural frequency of the pendulum is to push it once and then watch how it oscillates on its own. The frequency of that free oscillation will be the pendulum's resonance frequency which guarantees maximal amplitude in swinging with minimal driving push applied. If our pendulum is pushed with frequency equal or close to v_1, its amplitude will rise even with very light pushes. It is also easy to notice that if pushed at a different frequency, the amplitude will quickly decrease.

The concept of resonance in the biomechanics of locomotion has a long history (McMahon 1984). Resonance is widely recognized as useful for minimizing the energy cost of propelling body segments. Knowing how to tune into resonance is essential in acquiring skills and refining training in the martial arts and in sports like skating, tennis, and gymnastics. To match the limbs' natural frequencies, the motor control system regulates the moments of inertia of the limbs and changes the stiffness in the joints – thus tuning into resonance. During the swing phase of normal gait, the knee, hip, and elbow angles change the magnitude, depending on the speed of gait. This change in angle allows the leg to articulate with minimal muscle drive, at any given speed of gait (Lacquaniti et al. 2002; Stansfield et al. 2006).

5.5.2
Resonance in Running

In his short story *The New Accelerator*[3] published in 1943, H.G. Wells writes about a scientist, Professor Gibberne, who developed a drug which accelerated all processes in the human body. As the Professor explains to the narrator, "… you will be going several thousand times faster than you ever did before, heart, lungs, muscles, brain – everything – and you will hit hard without knowing it. You won't know it, you know. You'll feel just as you do now. Only everything in the world will seem to be going ever so many thousand times slower than it ever went before. That's what makes it so deuced queer."

In this fantastic story, the narrator and Professor Gibberne go for a walk after taking the newly developed drug. Their walk – and everything they see and do – appears to take a half an hour. But when they come back to the Professor's office, just when the drug's effects are wearing off, they see that their journey lasted for only a few seconds.

This great science fiction story challenges neuroscience with the nature of reaction time. Regarding the biomechanical probability of this extremely fast locomotion, the story is of course true fiction.

For example, the heroes were walking and running. These activities occur in the field of gravity, which is not affected by the *Accelerator* or any chemical agent. What can be affected by gravity are the ballistics of the body segments, when the frequencies of their oscillations are close to the natural frequencies of the segments. That closeness produces the effect of resonance, which minimizes the work of the muscles responsible for locomotion (Perry 1992). According to Eq. 5.9, when l_1 increases, the frequency v_1 decreases, and vice versa. The positioning of the rotating body's center of mass relative to the pivotal point defines its moment of inertia as a measure of the body's resistance to angular acceleration associated with oscillation. It is the analogue to mass as a measure of resistance to linear acceleration.

The moment of inertia I of a pendulum as a point mass m rotating about a known axis at a distance l_1 is defined by

$$I = ml_1^2 \qquad (5.10)$$

When a pendulum oscillates with its natural frequency, the resistance to the oscillation is minimal, while the pendulum resists being pushed at a faster or slower rate. The moment of inertia of a runner's thigh is determined by the distribution of mass of its tissues. Even

---

[3]The Complete Short Stories of H. G. Wells, St. Martins Press, Inc, New York, 1992

though the approximation of a thigh by a point mass is quite far from reality, we may use it to illuminate the difference in runners' anatomical features, which are better suited for running short or long distances.

Sprinters need legs capable of oscillating faster than the legs of long-distance runners, so they need to increase the natural frequency of their thigh (see Eq. 5.9), which corresponds to a smaller moment of inertia (see Eq. 5.10). To lower the moment of inertia, the center of mass has to be closer to the pivot. Thus, the closer the thigh's center of mass is to the hip joint, the lower its moment of inertia and the higher its natural frequency. That explains why sprinters bend their knees in the swing phase more than the long distant runners. That lowers the overall moment of inertia of the leg and allows it to oscillate faster relative to the hip joint.

To increase the leg's natural frequency, sprinters also work out to develop a cone-like thigh shape. For long-distance runners, the priority is endurance, which can be achieved by reducing the number of steps per time unit, that is, by reducing the natural frequency of the leg. Therefore, the moment of inertia of the segment has to be higher, and the thighs may be slimmer and have a more cylindrical shape.

Going back to Wells's story, we may now estimate how the heroes' thighs need to change in order to let them run hundreds of times faster than usual. According to Eq. 5.9, the required increase in natural frequency v_1 will diminish the distance l_1 from the pivot to the center of mass and the moment of inertia I in Eq. 5.10. Consequently, the entire mass of the thigh should be concentrated in the hip joint, while the rest of the segment should be a weightless rod.

5.5.3
When Resonance is Unwanted

We characterize gait as a sequence of coordinated restricted and unrestricted mobility in the body's joints. We believe that under this characterization, unrestricted mobility is no more important than restricted mobility. Rather, the opposite is true, considering the permanence of the task of preventing collapse due to gravity. This brings us to the assumption that there exists a mechanism that simultaneously controls both the tuning into, and also the tuning out of resonance. Since muscles perform the necessary restriction/fixation of joint articulation within the joint's range of motion, facilitating the muscles' efforts would minimize total muscle work.

Now, let us formulate a new task for the pendulum described in Sect. 5.5.1. Suppose that we know that the driving push continues to be applied with the resonance frequency v_1 determined above, but at this time we need to minimize the amplitude of the pendulum's swing. In other words, we would like to go out of resonance instead of going into resonance. One way to tune out of resonance is to change the natural frequency of the pendulum by changing its moment of inertia. It can be achieved by moving the bob up and down along the rod, which will change the value l_1 to l_2 or l_3. Let $l_2 < l_1 < l_3$. Then, according to Eq. 5.9, $v_2 > v_1 > v_3$.

The other way to tune out of resonance would be to enhance our model by including a resistance to swinging in the pivot. By changing the resistance, the natural frequency of the pendulum can be changed without changing the pendulum's length, but calculations are more complex.

The different tasks of tuning into and tuning out of resonance in human biomechanics can be seen in regular gait. During the stance phase, the foot of the weight-bearing leg is in contact with the ground. The stance phase lasts about 60% of the duration of each step. During the remaining 40% of the time required for a step, the leg is in *swing* phase, when the foot is in the air, translating forward. That translation can be approximated by the rotation of the leg in the hip joint, while the knee joint is bent up to 90°. There is a general agreement in biomechanics that utilizing the effect of resonance is a strategy of the human motion control system, since it minimizes energy expenditure and simplifies muscle control.

5.5.4
Spectral Optimization in Biomechanics of Locomotion

The human body can be modeled by a multi-linker, whose moments of inertia and natural frequencies have been calculated (McCronville et al. 1980). We suggested earlier (Pitkin 1989, 1992, 2010) that spectral analysis should be a part of the biomechanics of locomotion, similar to the role of the analysis of instability in rotor-shaft mechanisms (DeSmidt et al. 2002). As a consequence, optimization can be achieved by controlling only a few of the stiffnesses, similarly to mechanical systems.

Following Abramov (1983), we considered the biped gait of a poly-linker whose dynamics are described by a system of differential equations

$$Au'' + Bu' = Cu = f, \quad C = C\big(\lambda(t)\big) \tag{5.11}$$

where A, B, C are symmetric matrices of kinetic energy, dissipation, and potential energy, respectively, and $\lambda(t)$ is a controlled vector function of stiffnesses in the joints of the poly-linker.

We refer to studies where the stride has been divided based on the dominant mobility in metatarsal, ankle, and hip joints (Pitkin 1975; Hof et al. 1987; Pitkin 1991). In each of these phases, the human body is approximated by a system with one degree of freedom. Each of the allowed configurations has its own natural frequency ω^*, which prompts the body to tune into resonance-type mobility in one or a few joints. At the same time, the body must adjust its entire spectrum to assure that the joints, which have to be locked, are not affected by ω^*. In other words, ω^* is not only the resonantly advantageous frequency, but is also resonantly dangerous with respect to the integrity of the current body's configuration.

We will represent the human body by a system of stiffnesses $\lambda_1 \dots \lambda_9$, which correspond to the major anatomical joints (Fig. 5.14). We can see conflicting requirements of the stiffnesses, using as an example the hip joints with stiffnesses λ_2 and λ_3 when one leg is in stance phase and the other is in swing phase. That situation requires λ_2 to be adequate for the task of limiting mobility in the joint in order to prevent collapsing. In contrast, the stiffness λ_3 should not be an obstacle to free rotation of the forward leg. Thus, the stiffness λ_3 should be tuned into the resonance frequency of the leg oscillating at the hip joint, while the stiffness λ_2 should be tuned out of this frequency.

Let the transfer from one configuration to another be achieved by partially limiting the mobility in some joints having stiffnesses $\lambda_i(t)$. Then the problem of control over movement in the system can be substituted by a problem of control over its spectrum

Fig. 5.14 Model of changing body configurations by controlling stiffness in joints (Pitkin 2010)

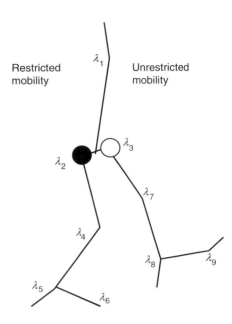

Restricted mobility

Unrestricted mobility

(Питкин 1984). For this we need to determine the possibility of tuning out the spectrum from the resonantly dangerous domain by varying the vector $\lambda(t)$, and to estimate how far it would be possible to tune out the spectrum of a pencil corresponding to (5.11).

That consideration reduces the problem of gait control mathematically to the problem of control over the spectrum of an operator pencil corresponding to the system of equations (5.11).

The mathematical problem was solved variationally in terms of abstract Rayleigh systems (Abramov 1983). To avoid the resonantly dangerous domain of the natural frequencies, the stiffnesses in joints for each phase of the stride have to be contained in corresponding intervals (Pitkin 1989).

The dual role of natural frequencies in human locomotion can be illustrated by the following example. During the stance period of gait, the ankle joint has to articulate freely for about 1/3 of a second (or with a frequency of 3.33 Hz), and then be fixed for the same duration (Perry 1992). The natural frequency of oscillation in a normal ankle joint is also 3.33 Hz (McCronville et al. 1980). Thus, during free articulation, the lower limb is tuned into resonance, and the subsequent fixation of the ankle joint, which is essential for the normal gait pattern, occurs in a resonantly dangerous zone. Stiffness in a joint depends on the balance between a resultant moment generated by the muscles causing rotation and resultant moment from the antagonist muscles that provide resistance to that rotation. There is no complete understanding of how the body control system solves this problem constantly. In the meantime, we would like to suggest the *principle of spectral reciprocity in locomotion* (Pitkin 2008) as follows:

"In locomotion, tuning into resonance to facilitate mobility in one group of joints is reciprocally associated with the tuning out of resonance to facilitate the restriction of mobility in other joints."

5.6
Conclusion

Understanding and appreciating the complexity and perfection of the biomechanical structure and control system of the human body is an important part of educating ourselves for the purpose of maintaining our health. Not knowing or ignoring the needs of the body can lead to serious negative consequences. As we demonstrated in this book, many problems are preventable if you incorporate the sanomechanical approach in your daily activities, transforming biomechanics as an academic discipline to *biomechanics for your life.*

References

Abe D, Yanagawa K et al (2004) Effects of load carriage, load position, and walking speed on energy cost of walking. Appl Ergon 35(4):329–335

Abramov YS (1983) Variational methods in the theory of operator pencils. Leningrad University Press, Leningrad

Antonsson EK, Mann RW (1985) The frequency content of gait. J Biomech 18(1):39–47

Aristotle (1934) The physics. Harvard University Press, Cambridge

Aristotle (1981) On the movement and progression of animals. Hildesheim, New York, Olms

Bernstein N (1967) The co-ordination and regulation of movements. Pergamon Press, Oxford

Breakey J (1976) Gait of unilateral below-knee amputees. Orth Prosth 30(4):17–24

Collins S, Ruina A et al (2005) Efficient bipedal robots based on passive-dynamic walkers. Science 307(5712):1082–1085

Czerniecki JM (1996) Rehabilitation in limb deficiency. 1. Gait and motion analysis. Arch Phys Med Rehabil 77(3 Suppl):S3–S8

Dankowicz H, Adolfsson J et al (2001) Repetitive gait of passive bipedal mechanisms in a three-dimensional environment. J Biomech Eng 123(1):40–46

DeSmidt HA, Wang KW et al (2002) Coupled torsion-lateral stability of a shaft-disk system driven through a universal joint. J Appl Mech 69(3):261–273

Dillingham TR, Lehmann JF et al (1992) Effect of lower limb on body propulsion. Arch Phys Med Rehabil 73(7):647–651

Elftman H (1938) The measurement of the external force in walking. Science 88:152–153

Elftman H (1939) Forces and energy changes in the leg during walking. Am J Physiol 125(2):339–356

Gage J (1990) An overview of normal walking. Instructional course lectures. Am Acad Orthop Surgeons 39:291–303

Gillespie KA, Dickey JP (2003) Determination of the effectiveness of materials in attenuating high frequency shock during gait using filterbank analysis. Clin Biomech (Bristol, Avon) 18(1):50–59

Goswami A, Espiau B et al (1996) Limit cycles and their stability in a passive bipedal gait. IEEE Int Conf Robot Automation 1:246–251

Hirsch R (2000) Seizing the light – a history of photography. McGraw-Hill, New-York

Hof AL, Geelen BA et al (1983) Calf muscle moment, work and efficiency in level walking; role of series elasticity. J Biomech 16(7):523–537

Hof AL, Pronk CN et al (1987) Comparison between EMG to force processing and kinetic analysis for the calf muscle moment in walking and stepping. J Biomech 20(2):167–178

Kadaba MP, Ramakrishnan HK et al (1990) Measurement of lower extremity kinematics during level walking. J Orthop Res 8(3):383–392

Kadaba MP, Ramakrishnan HK et al (1989) Repeatability of kinematic, kinetic, and electromyographic data in normal adult gait. J Orthop Res 7(6):849–860

Kepple TM, Siegel KL et al (1997) Relative contributions of the lower extremity joint moments to forward progression and support during gait. Gait Posture 6(1):1–8

Kerrigan DC, Todd MK et al (1998) Biomechanical gait alterations independent of speed in the healthy elderly: evidence for specific limiting impairments. Arch Phys Med Rehabil 79(3):317–322

Kirtley C (2005) Clinical gait analysis: theory and practice. Elsevier, Edinburgh; New York

Laaksonen MS, Kyrolainen H et al (2006) The association between muscle EMG and perfusion in knee extensor muscles. Clin Physiol Funct Imaging 26(2):99–105

Lacquaniti F, Ivanenko YP et al (2002) Kinematic control of walking. Arch Ital Biol 140(4):263–272

Lehmann JF, Price R et al (1993) Comprehensive analysis of dynamic elastic response feet: Seattle Ankle/Lite Foot versus SACH foot. Arch Phys Med Rehabil 74(8):853–861

Mann RA, Moran GT et al (1986) Comparative electromyography of the lower extremity in jogging, running, and sprinting. Am J Sports Med 14(6):501–510

May DR, Davis B (1974) Gait and the lower-limb amputee. Physiotherapy 60(6):166–171

McCronville J, Churchill T et al (1980) Anthropometric relationships of body and body segments moments of inertia. Anthropology Research Project, Inc., Yellow Springs

McGeer T (1990) Passive dynamic walking. Int J Rob Res 9(2):62–82

McMahon TA (1984) Muscles, reflexes, and locomotion. Princeton University Press, Princeton

Meglan D, Todd F (1994) Kinetics of human locomotion. In: Rose J, Gamble JG (eds) Human walking. Williams & Wilkins, Baltimore, pp 73–99

Meinders M, Gitter A et al (1998) The role of ankle plantar flexor muscle work during walking. Scand J Rehabil Med 30(1):39–46

Miura H, Shimoyama I (1984) Dynamic walk of a biped. Int J Rob Res 3(2):60–74

Mochon S, McMahon T (1979) Ballistic walking. An improved model. Math Biosci 52:241–260

Murray MP, Guten GN et al (1978) Function of the triceps surae during gait. Compensatory mechanisms for unilateral loss. J Bone Joint Surg Am 60(4):473–476

Oberg T, Karsznia A et al (1993) Basic gait parameters: reference data for normal subjects, 10–79 years of age. J Rehabil Res Dev 30(2):210–223

Perry J (1992) Gait analysis: normal and pathological function. Slack, Inc., Thorofare

Pitkin M (1975a) Kinematic and dynamic analysis of human gait (Rus). Proceedings of the first all-union conference in biomechanics, RNIITO, Riga, Latvia, 1995, pp 279–283

Pitkin M (1975b) Mechanics of the mobility of the human foot. Mech Solids 10(6):31–36

Pitkin M (1975c) Model of the foot with osseomorphic connection of its elements. Prostheses Prosthet, Moscow 35:83–89

Pitkin M (1977) Human foot as a propulsor in gait. Prostheses Prosthet, Moscow 42:34–39

Pitkin M (1984) Simulation of a foot contribution in ballistic knee extension. Prostheses Prosthet, Moscow 70:98–102

Pitkin M (1989) Tuning out of resonance during walking and requirements for footwear. Proceedings of the XII international congress of biomechanics, Los Angeles, CA, 1989, pp 336–337

Pitkin M (1991) New stride phases and the development of sport shoe prototype to assist the calf muscles during heel-off. Proceedings of the 15th annual meeting, American Society of Biomechanics, Tempe, Arizona, 1991, pp 266–267

Pitkin M (1992) Mathematical criterion of tuning out of resonance and its application in human locomotion. Proceedings of the second international conference on biomathematics, The Republica di San Marino, 1992

Pitkin M (1995) Mechanical outcome of a rolling joint prosthetic foot, and its performance in dorsiflexion phase of the trans-tibial amputee gait. J Prosthet Orthot 7(4):114–123

Pitkin M (1997) Pain preventive gait synergy hypothesis in leg amputees. Proceedings of the XVIth congress of the ISB, Tokyo, Japan, 1997

Pitkin M (2006a) Biomechanics of the joints' moments in design of the lower limb prostheses. Bull Russ Guild Prosthetists Orthotists 11(1(23)):27–33

Pitkin M (2006b) Propulsion function of the foot as a component of ballistic synergy of gait. Bull Russ Guild Prosthetists Orthotists 11(3-4/25-26):38–43

Pitkin M (2008) Principle of spectral reciprocity in biomechanics of locomotion and rehabilitation. Open Rehabil J 1(4):1–4

Pitkin M (2009) Regular and intentional generation of propulsion in normal gait as prototype for prosthetic design. IEEE Eurocon 2009 international conference, St. Petersburg, Russia, 18–23 May 2009

Pitkin MR (2010) Biomechanics of lower limb prosthetics. Springer, Heidelberg

Rab GT (1994) Muscle: human walking. Williams & Wilkins, Baltimore

Riley PO, Della Croce U et al (2001) Propulsive adaptation to changing gait speed. J Biomech 34(2):197–202

Rose J, Gamble JG (eds) (1994) Human walking. Williams & Wilkins, Baltimore

Rosenberg RM (1991) Analytical dynamics of discrete systems. Plenum Press, New York

Rossi SA, Doyle W et al (1995) Gait initiation of persons with below-knee amputation: the characterization and comparison of force profiles. J Rehabil Res Dev 32(2):120–127

Saunders JB, Inman VT et al (1953) The major determinants in normal and pathological gait. J Bone Joint Surg Am 35-A(3):543–558

Simon SR (2004) Quantification of human motion: gait analysis-benefits and limitations to its application to clinical problems. J Biomech 37(12):1869–1880

Skinner HB, Effeney DJ (1985) Gait analysis in amputees. Am J Phys Med 64(2):82–89

Spiegel MR, Liu J (2001) Mathematical handbook of formulas and tables. McGraw-Hill

Stansfield BW, Hillman SJ et al (2006) Regression analysis of gait parameters with speed in normal children walking at self-selected speeds. Gait Posture 23(3):288–294

Sutherland DH (1966) An electromyographic study of the plantar flexors of the ankle in normal walking on the level. J Bone Joint Surg Am 48(1):66–71

Sutherland DH, Cooper L et al (1980a) The role of the ankle plantar flexors in normal walking. J Bone Joint Surg Am 62(3):354–363

Sutherland DH, Olshen R et al (1980b) The development of mature gait. J Bone Joint Surg Am 62(3):336–353

Tseng SC, Liu W et al (2006) Muscle activation profiles about the knee during Tai-Chi stepping movement compared to the normal gait step. J Electromyogr Kinesiol 17(3):372–380

Watanabe H, Urabe K et al (2010) Quality of life, knee function, and physical activity in Japanese elderly women with early-stage knee osteoarthritis. J Orthop Surg Hong Kong 18(1):31–34

Weber WE, Weber E (1836) Die Mechanik Der Menschlichen Gerverzeuge. English edition: Weber WE, Weber E (1991) Mechanics of the human walking apparatus (trans. Maquet P and Furlong R). Springer-Verlag, Berlin

Winter DA (1979) Biomechanics of human movement. John Wiley & Sons, Inc., New York

Winter DA (1983) Energy generation and absorption at the ankle and knee during fast, natural, and slow cadence. Clin Orthop Relat Res 175:147–154

Yamaguchi J, Kinoshita N, et al (1996) Development of a dynamic biped walking system for humanoid – development of a BipedWalking robot adapting to the humans' living floor. IEEE international conference on robotics and automation, Anchorage, 1996, pp 232–239

Zajac FE, Neptune RR et al (2003) Biomechanics and muscle coordination of human walking: part II: lessons from dynamical simulations and clinical implications. Gait Posture 17(1):1–17

Богданов, В. А. and В. С. Гурфинкель (1976) Биомеханика локомоций человека. - В кн.: Физиология движений. Л., Наука

Морейнис, И. Ш., Г. П. Гриценко, et al. (1971). "Биомеханический анализ ходьбы в норме и на протезах." Протезирование и протезостроение, сб. трудов, вып. XXVI, М., ЦНИИПП: 7–16

Питкин, М. Р. (1975). "Модель стопы с остеоморфным соединением элементов." Протезирование и протезостроение, сб. трудов вып. 35, М., ЦНИИПП: 83–89

Питкин, М. Р. (1977). Стопа человека как движитель при ходьбе. Протезирование и протезостроение, сб. трудов вып. 42, М., ЦНИИПП: 34–39

Питкин, М. Р. (1980). "Математическое моделирование ходьбы." Клиническая биомеханика // Под ред. В.И. Филатова. - Л.: Медицина: 74–82

Питкин, М. Р. (1984). Управление движением многозвенника как проблема управления спектром операторного пучка. Материалы III Всесоюзн. совещания по робото-техн. системам. Воронеж, 4, 66–67

Питкин, М. Р. (1985). Кинематические и динамические характеристики ходьбы в зависимости от фрикционных свойств опорной поверхности. Протезирование и протезостроение, сб. трудов вып. 73, М., ЦНИИПП: 98–102

Sanomechanics for Respiration

6

The exercises discussed in previous chapters were meant to promote hydraulic connectivity in the skeleton. Capillarity was the mechanism responsible for transporting the synovial fluid. In this chapter, we will examine some biomechanical aspects of respiration that depend on other mechanisms for transporting liquids in the body. Specifically, we will discuss the connection between breathing and swallowing. Familiarity with the natural mechanics of how airways are cleared will help us consciously prevent common problems associated with breathing.

6.1
Nasal Polyps

My interest in the biomechanics of how airways are cleared goes back to 2004 when I was diagnosed with nasal polyps. They blocked my nasal airways completely; I could not sleep and my throat was painfully dry because I could only breathe through my mouth. Surgery for polyps removal was scheduled at my request, but I canceled it after a conversation with a friend who had undergone a similar procedure earlier. He told me that he was in pain for ten days after surgery, and that in five years he had to have surgery again since the polyps returned. I would have agreed to tolerate the postoperative pain, but the knowledge that the procedure may need to be repeated forced me to think more about the problem.

In attempts to explain what caused the polyps to develop I recalled my flight from Beijing to Boston two weeks before. During the 14-h flight, my nose became congested. As people usually do, I worked hard with tissues, and frankly, with very little success. "I might have worked too hard" – this was the thought that came to my mind now. I suspected that the mechanical loads associated with the frequent forced exhalation on the plane exceeded some limitations for the recovery of the epithelial tissues in the nose. A visual confirmation for this hypothesis came in a restroom of the Tufts University Medical Center, when my hands were under the dryer (Fig. 6.1a). What I saw were waves of skin appearing under the influence of a strong airflow (Fig. 6.1b).

Later, I found in the literature some arguments in favor of the hypothesis that a strong airflow in the nasal cavity may be responsible for the polyps' development. There were reports on the extremely complex nature and delicate structure of the liquid–epithelium system, rendering it susceptible to surface tension–induced injury (Elad and Schroter 2008; Ghadiali and Gaver 2008).

M.R. Pitkin, *Biomechanics for Life*,
DOI: 10.1007/978-3-642-17177-2_6, © Springer-Verlag Berlin Heidelberg 2011

Fig. 6.1 Development of
skin waves on a hand (**a**)
with airflow from the hand
dryer (**b**)

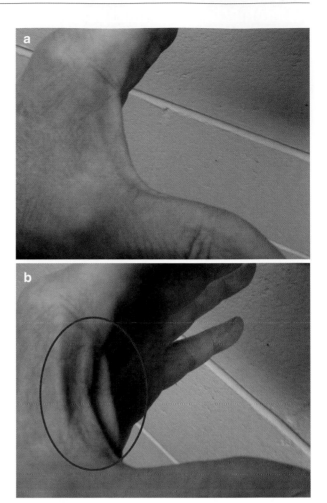

The next step was to effectively reopen my airways without surgery. I will tell you here
what I did and why. The effect of my practices was that at my checkup in six months, the
doctor didn't find any polyps.

6.2
Pathway of Air

Air, as well as water and food enter the throat, where their routes diverge. Air enters
the *trachea* and water and food pass into the *esophagus* (Fig. 6.2). To prevent water
and food from entering the lungs, there is a valve called the *epiglottis,* which closes
the entrance to the trachea when needed. The trachea is lined with epithelial cells
which produce *mucus*. The mucus traps inhaled foreign particles, and then transports

Fig. 6.2 Air (*blue arrows*) passages through nasal and/ or oral cavity controlled by the epiglottis. Orange arrows show passage of mucus and food and/or saliva via swallowing

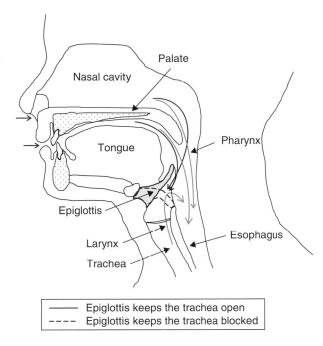

	Epiglottis keeps the trachea open
- - - -	Epiglottis keeps the trachea blocked

them to the *larynx*, and then the *pharynx* (Fig. 6.2). It can then either be swallowed or expelled by coughing *as phlegm. Motile cilia,* which are protuberances that project from the epithelium cells (Fig. 6.3), transport the mucus.

Normally, the signal to swallow the mucus is reflexive. The need to cough arises when large objects, like a piece of food, are inhaled, or when the production of mucus is increased as a means to address infection or irritation.

Fighting an infection or the hot smoke and particles from cigarettes results in greater mucus viscosity, making it more difficult for the motile cilia to transport the mucus along the trachea for further removal. Slower delivery of mucus to the pharynx compromises the effectiveness of the swallowing reflex. The control system "doesn't know" about the increased volume of mucus in the trachea and in the lungs. But the control system "knows" about the decreased level of oxygen in the blood as a result of the mechanical obstacles to airflow. This triggers a coughing reflex, as a backup measure to continue breathing and increase its effectiveness.

The mechanics of swallowing are such that when the pharynx contracts, its contents move down to the esophagus, bypassing the trachea which is blocked by the epiglottis (Fig. 6.2). The back end of the *palate* blocks the entrance of air through the nose; the closed lips block the entrance of the air through the mouth. This forms an effective biological pump.

Like with any pump (Beitler SR, Lindahl EJ (1953); Butler E (1922)), a zone with positive pressure and a zone with negative pressure are created. In our case, the positive pressure under the pharynx causes the pharynx's contents to move down to the esophagus. The swallowed matter is not in free fall toward the stomach, but is driven by coordinated wave-like contractions and relaxations called *peristalsis*. The first contraction of the esophagus takes place above the swallowed matter, but below the epiglottis. That tells the valves to

Fig. 6.3 Scanning electron microscopy micrograph of the motile cilia projecting from respiratory epithelium (photograph by Charles Daghlian, adopted with permission)

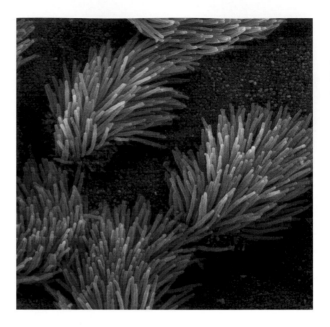

open the larynx's entrance to the trachea and the palate's entrance to the nasal cavity (Fig. 6.2). These coordinated actions produce a zone of negative pressure, which encompasses the trachea and the nasal cavity.

The negative pressure attracts and moves the mucus from the trachea and the nasal cavity to the area of the pharynx. This constitutes the second mechanism of clearing the airways and compliments the work of motile cilia (Fig. 6.3).

This also explains why drinking water may help in suppressing a cough. The additional cycles of swallowing prompted by drinking helps in the removal of the extra volume of mucus from the trachea. When it is removed, the airflow pathway widens, and the physical need for coughing is reduced.

6.3
Sanomechanics for Breathing

A more powerful pump for transporting the mucus to the pharynx for further swallowing is the diaphragm and the accessory (intercostal) muscles of respiration, in the period between inhalation and exhalation. The longer this period, the more efficiently the airways will be cleared.

Why should the length of the period matter? The "waiting" period between inhalation and exhalation is the time when the motile cilia work most efficiently, and when the negative pressure pumping the mucus into the trachea and the nasal cavity is established. Let us talk about this mechanism in greater detail.

Fig. 6.4 The middle and posterior mediastina with diaphragm (adopted from Gray and Lewis (1918) with permission from Bartleby. com, Inc.)

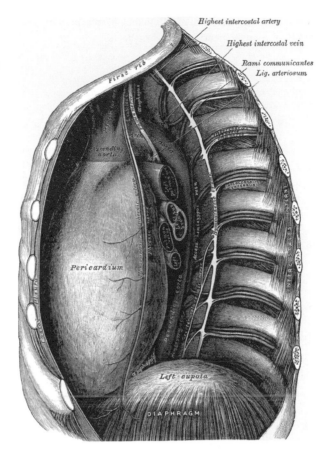

When the cupola of the diaphragm contracts, it flattens, the contents of the abdomen are moved downward, and the thoracic volume increases (Fig. 6.4). This creates negative pressure inside the thorax relative to atmospheric pressure, which pushes the outside air into the lungs.

In the process of regular exhalation, the accessory muscles first relax, and then the cupola of the relaxed diaphragm moves up (Fig. 6.4). That increases the pressure in the thorax and expels air from the lungs. The process stops when the pressure inside the thorax equals the atmospheric pressure outside. Such breathing does not stimulate the transport of mucus.

When we consciously expel air, and exhalation is active, the abdominal muscles assist in the exhalation. The thoracic volume then reaches its absolute minimum, which allows inhalation to be more active, and more new air to enter the lungs. If we hold our breath after exhaling actively and then relax the abdominal muscles, the volume of the thorax increases and the pressure inside becomes lower than the atmospheric pressure. Since the pressure in the epithelial cells is atmospheric, a pressure difference is developed between the inside and outside of the cell's membrane. The pressure difference activates secretion from the cells, delivering more water to the mucus on the walls of trachea and nasal cavity. Mucus moves up along the trachea, and downward from the nasal cavity to the pharynx.

The increased quantity of matter in the pharynx area triggers the swallowing reflex, and we swallow, thereby clearing the airways.

6.4
Conclusion

As soon as I realized why holding my breath after actively exhaling facilitates swallowing and leads to an effective clearing of the airways, I began practicing this technique along with the autosuggestion: "My nasal cavities become clearer with each swallow." I sensed how my airways were opening, bringing relief and encouraging me to continue. While there is no direct relation to the floating skeleton concept here, the combination of creating the exercise with understanding its biomechanics and with the corresponding autosuggestion and positive feedback is indeed *sanomechanics* by definition.

References

Beitler SR, Lindahl EJ (1953) Hydraulic machinery. Ronald, New York, Ronald Press Co
Butler E (1922) Modern pumping and hydraulic machinery as applied to all purposes, with explanation of the theoretical principles involved, construction, working, and relative advantages. Being a practical handbook for engineers, designers, and others. C. Griffin & Company Ltd., London
Elad D, Schroter RC (2008) Respiratory biomechanics. Respir Physiol Neurobiol 163(1–3):1–2
Ghadiali SN, Gaver DP (2008) Biomechanics of liquid-epithelium interactions in pulmonary airways. Respir Physiol Neurobiol 163(1–3):232–243
Gray H, Lewis WH (1918) Anatomy of the human body. Lea & Febiger, Philadelphia, Bartleby.com, 2000. www.bartleby.com/1-7/

Postface

In Sophocles's (497–406 BC) tragedy *Oedipus Rex* (Sophocles 2007), when the Priest thanks Oedipus:

> "For you came here, to our Cadmeian city,
> and freed us from the tribute we were paying
> to that *cruel singer*—and yet you knew
> no more than we did and had not been taught"[1]

he is referring to Oedipus's intellectual victory over the Sphinx (the *cruel singer*). The Sphinx, a creature with a lion's body, wings, and head and torso of a woman, tyrannized the citizens of Thebes by not allowing anyone passage into or out of the city, unless the traveler could answer the riddle: "What walks on four legs in the morning, two legs at noon, and three legs in the evening?"

Oedipus solved the riddle, the Sphinx committed suicide, and the city was saved. The correct answer, discovered by Oedipus, was "a human being." In a man's early ages he crawls on all fours, and in his old age man uses a cane as the third leg.

Traditionally, Oedipus has been treated as a hero, and his conquest over the Sphinx has been regarded as a symbol of the triumph of light over darkness (Breal 2010). I too prize Oedipus's courage and clever thinking, but refuse to see "three-legged" walking as an inevitable attribute of elderly people. I believe that timely care of the skeleton's health can effectively fight with pain from walking that we begin to feel as we age.

By saying "timely" with relation to "care" it might be useful to recall a story about the *Fisherman and the Jinnee (Genie)* told in the *Tales from the Thousand and One Nights*. When one day the fisherman hurled his net far out into the sea, and brought it back to land, he found in it a bottle. Once he opened the bottle, there burst from it a great column of smoke which resolved itself into a jinnee with his head touching the clouds, while his feet were planted in the sand. The fisherman expected that the jinnee would rightfully reward him for freeing him from his imprisonment. The opposite came true. The jinnee announced that he will kill the fisherman, and gave his explanations as follows:

> "In the ocean depth I vowed: 'I will bestow eternal riches on him who sets me free!' But a hundred years passed away and no one freed me. In the second hundred years of my imprisonment I said: 'For him who frees me I will open up the buried treasures of the earth!' And yet no one freed me. Whereupon I flew into a rage and swore: 'I will kill the

---

[1]Courtesy of the Publisher

M.R. Pitkin, *Biomechanics for Life*,
DOI: 10.1007/978-3-642-17177-2, © Springer-Verlag Berlin Heidelberg 2011

man who sets me free, allowing him only to choose the manner of his death!" Now it was you who set me free; therefore prepare to die and choose the way that I shall kill you."[2]

The rest of the story is devoted to the fisherman's successful strategy of surviving and to making the jinnee his loyal servant. What I would like to take from this passage is the timeless message that even right things, if done too late, can lead to unwanted consequences.

Whenever a joint becomes too painful, due to its isolation from the hydraulic net (as described in the *Floating Skeleton* concept in Chap. 1), I suggest to myself the image of the jinnee trapped in that joint. I tell myself: "Do sanomechanics exercises (Chap. 4) now. Free the jinnee while he will still serve me happily."

Now, in the end, I would like to salute you, my reader, who may have discovered in this book new ways of improving your health. I hope that you were skeptical enough to be interested in the scientific facts and hypotheses behind the approach here called sanomechanics. If the arguments were reasonably convincing and you will consider applying this approach to your daily life, I see my mission as accomplished, as one more person will benefit from the findings which were helpful for me.

References

Breal, M. Le Myth D'Oedipe (2010). Whitefish, MO, Kessinger Publishing Company
Sophocles. (2007) Oedipus the King (Translated by Ian Johnston). Richer Resources Publications, Arlington Tales of the Thousand and One Nights (translated by N.J. Dawood (1973)). Penguin Book, London

[2]Courtesy of the Publisher